AF606474

PREGNANCY AND INFANTS: MEDICAL, PSYCHOLOGICAL AND SOCIAL ISSUES SERIES

HUMAN PLACENTA: STRUCTURE AND DEVELOPMENT, CIRCULATION AND FUNCTIONS

PREGNANCY AND INFANTS: MEDICAL, PSYCHOLOGICAL AND SOCIAL ISSUES SERIES

Focus on Milk and Infants
Viroj Wiwanitkit
2009. ISBN: 978-1-60741-106-2

Infectious Pregnancy Complications
Richard N. Canfield (Editor)
2009. ISBN: 978-1-60471-038-6

Drugs During Pregnancy
Bengt Källén
2009. ISBN: 978-1-60876-154-8

Breastfeeding: Methods, Benefits to the Infant and Mother, and Difficulties
Wilma G. Nueland (Editor)
2010. ISBN: 978-1-60741-933-4

Nonmarital Childbearing: Trends, Reasons and Policy
Gilberto de la Rayes (Editor)
2010. ISBN: 978-1-60741-756-9

Human Placenta: Structure and Development, Circulation and Functions
Eirik Berven and Andras Freberg (Editors)
2010. ISBN: 978-1-60876-457-0

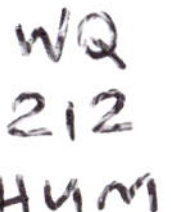
WQ
212
HUM

Imperial College London
2407439036

Imperial College
London

the Library
www.imperial.ac.uk/library

THREE WEEK LOAN (STANDARD)
Please return or renew by the due date.
Fines may be charged on items returned late.

- 1 FEB 2013
- 6 DEC 2013
2 6 JAN 2016

PREGNANCY AND INFANTS: MEDICAL, PSYCHOLOGICAL AND SOCIAL ISSUES SERIES

HUMAN PLACENTA: STRUCTURE AND DEVELOPMENT, CIRCULATION AND FUNCTIONS

EIRIK BERVEN
AND
ANDRAS FREBERG
EDITORS

Nova Biomedical Books
New York

Copyright © 2010 by Nova Science Publishers, Inc.

All rights reserved. No part of this book may be reproduced, stored in a retrieval system or transmitted in any form or by any means: electronic, electrostatic, magnetic, tape, mechanical photocopying, recording or otherwise without the written permission of the Publisher.

For permission to use material from this book please contact us:
Telephone 631-231-7269; Fax 631-231-8175
Web Site: http://www.novapublishers.com

NOTICE TO THE READER

The Publisher has taken reasonable care in the preparation of this book, but makes no expressed or implied warranty of any kind and assumes no responsibility for any errors or omissions. No liability is assumed for incidental or consequential damages in connection with or arising out of information contained in this book. The Publisher shall not be liable for any special, consequential, or exemplary damages resulting, in whole or in part, from the readers' use of, or reliance upon, this material.

Independent verification should be sought for any data, advice or recommendations contained in this book. In addition, no responsibility is assumed by the publisher for any injury and/or damage to persons or property arising from any methods, products, instructions, ideas or otherwise contained in this publication.

This publication is designed to provide accurate and authoritative information with regard to the subject matter covered herein. It is sold with the clear understanding that the Publisher is not engaged in rendering legal or any other professional services. If legal or any other expert assistance is required, the services of a competent person should be sought. FROM A DECLARATION OF PARTICIPANTS JOINTLY ADOPTED BY A COMMITTEE OF THE AMERICAN BAR ASSOCIATION AND A COMMITTEE OF PUBLISHERS.

Library of Congress Cataloging-in-Publication Data

Available upon request

ISBN: 978-1-60876-457-0

Published by Nova Science Publishers, Inc. ✢ New York

Contents

Preface

The placenta is a fetomaternal organ provided by nature to aid development of the growing embryo by facilitating gas and nutrient exchange between the mother and fetus and by helping to maintain fetomaternal tolerance. Aside from playing an age-old and essential role in fetal development, placental tissues have also attracted the interest of clinical scientists due to their potential utility as a therapeutic agent. This book provides an overview of the clinical applications which have been described for placental tissue or are currently applied, as well as a summary of the most recent results obtained in preclinical studies, which present promising perspectives for the future clinical application of these cells. The trophoblast, a cell type of the placenta, is also outlined in this book, as well as its function in the placenta during pregnancy and its role in developmental processes and gynecological diseases. In addition, pregnancy-specific glycoproteins (PSGs) are secreted proteins which are produced by the rodent and primate placenta, and play a critical role in pregnancy success. This book summarizes and analyzes the data on structure and function of PSGs known to date. Relatively recent data of PSG-derived biologically active peptides are also described. Other chapters examine placental functions and their role in predicting development and disease in infancy and childhood, and the role of insulin like growth factors (IFGs) in normal and abnormal placental and fetal development during pregnancy.

Chapter I - The placenta is a fetomaternal organ provided by nature to aid development of the growing embryo by facilitating gas and nutrient exchange between the mother and fetus and by helping to maintain fetomaternal tolerance. Aside from playing an age-old and essential role in fetal development, placental tissues have also attracted the interest of clinical scientists due to their potential utility as a therapeutic agent.

For decades, the human term placenta, which is available in plentiful supply and raises no ethical concerns for its procurement, has been used as a surgical material in skin transplantation, as a biological dressing for treatment of skin wounds, burn injuries and chronic leg ulcers, for prevention of tissue adhesion in surgical procedures, and in ocular surface reconstruction.

More recently, human placenta has also attracted increasing attention from cell and molecular biologists, who have turned to this tissue in the search for a novel stem cell source. Indeed, cells derived from the amniotic and chorionic fetal membranes have been shown to present with high plasticity and to possess low immunogenicity as well as immunomodulatory properties, thereby making them prime candidates for development of cell therapy-based tissue regeneration strategies.

This chapter will provide an overview of the clinical applications which have been described for placental tissue or which are currently applied, and will also give a summary of the most recent results obtained in preclinical studies, which present promising perspectives for the future clinical application of placenta-derived cells.

Chapter II - The placenta, which is a temporary organ derived from the fetus, is removed after delivery. This organ is critical to support fetus development via optimal regulation between mother and fetus. The placenta includes different cell types: amnion, trophoblast, decidual cells, Hofbauer cells, endothelium, and mesenchymal cells. Among these cell types, the trophoblast is one of the earliest to differentiate and shows an extensive proliferation or/and differentiation up to the formation of the normal placenta as a major cell population. The characterization of the trophoblast shows dynamic changes according to placental development during pregnancy. This brief review outlines the development of the trophoblast and its function in the placenta during pregnancy. The authors review how the trophoblast can play a role in developmental processes under various environment factors and link this function to gynecological diseases. Finally, the authors introduce the latest research in trophoblast differentiation and the therapeutic potential of trophoblast stem cells for obstetrical and gynecological diseases.

Chapter III - The placenta plays a major role in regulating fetal growth and development during human pregnancy. The placental development correlates with the fetal growth. Insulin like growth factors (IGF-1 and -2) are essential growth factors promoting cellular multiplication for growth and differentiation of the placental and fetal tissues. Placenta is a major source of IGFs during pregnancy. In addition, IGF-binding proteins (BP -1, -3 and -4) and metalloproteinase enzymes (pregnancy associated plasma protein A; PAPP-A and A Disintegrin and Metalloproteinase 12s; ADAM-12s) are abundantly produced and are quantifiable in maternal sera during pregnancy. The levels of these factors in maternal sera vary with the progression of normal pregnancy, and may be reduced in various adverse pregnancy conditions. It is suggested that the placenta contributes to IGF production and its biosynthesis is regulated by the "IGF-axis" involving growth hormone releasing factor ghrelin (GHRL) and a structurally variant growth hormone (GH-2) during pregnancy. Unlike production of IGFs during the postnatal period which is an endocrine process with the participation of the hypothalamus, pituitary and liver, generation of IGFs during the prenatal periods to a large extent is by paracrine-autocrine processes. The placenta and fetal membranes produce IGF-binding proteins (IGF-BPs) and metalloproteinases (PAPP-A and ADAM-12s) and active and free IGFs are generated by proteolytic separation of IGFs and BPs. Availability of free IGFs which may bind with its cellular receptors for multiplication and differentiation of cells is required for prenatal development. PAPP-A is released in plasma as a complex of proform of eosinophil major basic protein (pro-MBP). The proteolytic activity of PAPP-A is presumably regulated by binding with pro-MBP which inhibits its proteinase activity. A variety of genes associated with these factors are expressed in placental and other conceptus tissues and their relative expression (mRNA and proteins) may be related to adverse pregnancy outcomes. In addition, single nucleotide polymorphisms (SNPs) and mutations which are variations of nucleotide sequences of genes may affect the functions of cells and differentiation and development of the fetus and placenta. Thus, both biosynthesis and bioavailability of IGFs may play a critical role in normal and abnormal placental and fetal development during pregnancy, and associated with the adverse outcomes, including intrauterine fetal growth retardation (IUGR) and premature births which significantly influence neonatal survival and morbidity, and subsequent postnatal life.

Chapter IV - Pregnancy-specific glycoproteins (PSGs) are secreted proteins which are produced by the rodent and primate placenta and play a critical role in pregnancy success. Genes which encode PSGs belong to carcinoembryonic antigen (CEA) gene family, which is included in immunoglobulin (Ig) gene superfamily. In humans, to date there are 11 protein products of these genes which are designated as PSG1–11. In rodents there are 17 PSGs, which are designated as PSG16–32. Human PSGs were first discovered in serum of pregnant women and were initially named as trophoblast-specific beta globulins (TBGs). Little later they were isolated from placental extracts and also revealed in serum of patients with trophoblastic tumors. Biological role of PSGs is not fully elucidated to date. However a number of experimental data and clinical observations allow supposing their critical role in the maintenance of pregnancy. Low PSG levels in the maternal circulation are associated with threatened abortions, intrauterine retardation and fetal hypoxia.

It has been shown that PSGs function as immunomodulatory proteins which regulate activity of T-lymphocytes and secretion of cytokines by monocytes and macrophages. Also, PGSs may participate in maternal vasculature remodeling through influencing on secretion of pro-angiogenic agents such as transforming growth factor-beta-1 (TGF-β1) and vascular endothelial growth factor (VEGF) by different cell types involved in the development of placenta.

Several functional domains have been described in PSG structures. For example, tripeptide RGD has been revealed in N-terminal immunoglobulin (Ig)-like domain of most of human PSGs. It is proposed that RGD motif of PSGs is involved in binding to integrin receptors. Binding of mouse PSGs to integrin-associated receptor CD9 has been demonstrated. In the author's laboratory some human PSG-derived oligopeptide fragments have been shown to possess biological activity. This chapter is devoted to summarizing and analyzing of data on structure and function of PSGs known to date. Also, relatively recent data of PSG-derived biologically active peptides are described.

Chapter V - Thrombosis and thromboembolism of various etiology, which are conditioned by activation of blood clotting factors and of fibrin stabilizing factor (FXIIIa) especially, are among the most severe and widespread kinds of blood-clotting pathologies. The last one catalyzes formation of γ-glutamyl-ε-lysin cross link reactions at the sites of α- and γ-polypeptide chains of fibrin molecules. For there are no physiologic inhibitors of FXIIIa, uncontrolled elevation of its enzymatic activity leads to hyper stability of thrombus to plasmin hydrolysis and makes fibrinolytic therapy ineffective. This fact determines importance to search ways of FXIIIa transpeptidase activity regulation using various approaches from outside. The ability of cysteine proteinase inhibitors (CPIs) isolated from tubers of potato (Solanum tuberosum L.) to suppress transpeptidase activity of fibrin stabilizing factor (FXIIIa) through the direct effect on the essential SH group of the enzyme active site has been studied. The formation of fibrin clots soluble in 5 M urea and 2% acetic acid as well as spectrophotometric turbidity analysis of the stabilization and resistance of fibrin clots formed in the presence of FXIIIa and CPIs from potato tubers to plasmin, and electrophoresis of reduced fibrin and casein samples indicate the decrease or absence of covalent cross-linking of fibrin and casein chains. In addition, CPIs added to the substrate proved to decelerate fibrinogen polymerization almost twice relative to control. It is concluded that natural CPIs can both take part in the regulation of FXIIIa transpeptidase activity *in vitro* and modify the substrate.

Chapter VI - Factor XIIIa plays an important role in stabilization of fibrin clot formed during blood coagulation. Recent reports indicate that factor XIIIa influence formation of coated platelets, which have high procoagulant activity and retain on their surface high levels of alphagranule proteins, express surface phosphatidylserine after platelet activation. It was also discovered that new cysteine proteinase inhibitors (CPIs) from potato could take regulate factor XIIIa transglutaminase activity. The aim of the present study was to determine the effect of CPIs on coated platelets formation during platelet activation and on enzyme activities in blood coagulation. The authors found that CPIs decreased the coated platelets subpopulation dose-dependently. They reduced thrombin generation by nearly 40 % both in platelet-rich plasma and in plateletpoor plasma as compared with control, and dose-dependently decreased activity of factor Xa and thrombin. In conclusion, the obtained data show that cysteine proteinase inhibitors have influence on platelet and plasma components of blood coagulation, and suggest that further purification and characterization of these inhibitors are of practical significance and interest.

Chapter VII - Placenta and fetus are closely linked in the so-called feto-placental unit. Therefore, the placenta contains information of intrauterine fetal life. This information might be of relevance for future processes in the then independent human organism. There are two principle ways of getting access to placental endocrine function with relevance for the fetus. More indirectly, during pregnancy serological maternal examinations e.g. of angiogenetic factors may help to predict the risk of evolving preeclampsia and possible secondary fetal involvement. However, direct access to the fetal side of the feto-placental unit is more difficult without injury at least during pregnancy. After delivery there is easy availability of placental samples, allowing for the analysis of feto-placental endocrinology and potential prediction of future developments arising from these conditions. The authors are currently conducting a multicenter study to predict the probability of later disease inflicted by a hostile intrauterine environment. An early prediction of risk of future disease would help to initiate early preventive measures.

Chapter VIII - The renin-angiotensin system (RAS) is one of main regulators of blood pressure and electrolyte balance during pregnancy. All the components of the RAS have been reported to be expressed in the utero-placental unit. Angiotensin (Ang) II is increasingly recognized as a growth factor, both in its own right and through interactions with other growth factors. Ang II synthesized in the placenta may serve as an autocrine/paracrine modulator of placental function. In addition to its role in regulation of blood pressure during normal pregnancy, Ang II is suggested to be involved in regulation of placentation through regulation of trophoblast invasion, angiogenesis and placental vascular development. These key effects of Ang II, in addition to its capacity to induce inflammatory response, suggest that increased vascular sensitivity to Ang II may have an important role in the increase in vascular resistance and elevated blood pressure seen pregnancy complications such as intra-uterin growth retardation (IUGR) and preeclampsia. Magnesium sulfate ($MgSO_4$) is used in pregnancy as either prophylaxis/treatment for eclamptic seizures or for preterm labor tocolysis. The author's group has shown that $MgSO_4$ may attenuate Ang II induced placental vasoconstriction, and may affect Ang II induced placental cytokine production. This review summarizes the current understanding of the physiological aspects of Ang II in the utero-placental unit and its role in the pathogenesis of pregnancy disorders such as preeclampsia. Furthermore, the possible interactions between Ang II and $MgSO_4$ in the placental unit are also discussed.

Chapter IX - The differentiation process and cell-cell fusion of human trophoblasts in the human placenta are controlled by a variety of regulatory genes and key molecules. In this article, the authors focus on the fusogenic glycoprotein syncytin-1, which originally derived from the human endogenous retrovirus HERV-W. In addition, the authors look at its transcription factor GCMa (glial cells missing-a or Gcm1).

The authors propose that GCMa-driven syncytin-1 expression is a key mechanism for syncytiotrophoblast formation in the human placenta. Besides the physiological significance of syncytin-1 and GCMa, the authors discuss their pathophysiological role in pre-eclampsia and intrauterine growth restriction (IUGR). In addition, the authors focus on the effects of hypoxia on the expression of syncytin-1 and GCMa in trophoblastic cells because changing oxygen availability contributes to abnormal placental development. Basically, any alteration of the cAMP signaling cascade involving protein kinase A (PKA), GCMa and syncytin-1 can be considered a major risk factor for diminished trophoblast differentiation and impaired syncytiotrophoblast formation, followed by placental dysfunction, for example, in the course of hypoxia. Furthermore, hypoxia-related down-regulation of syncytin-1 can, to a great extent, be compensated by stimulating the cAMP-driven PKA pathway. Considering that pre-eclampsia is unique to humans and that syncytin-1 is derived from the HERV-W family exclusively found in humans and in higher primates, syncytin-1 is an interesting candidate for research into human placental physiology and altered placental function.

Similarly, the authors describe a putative mode of action at the cellular level. Using a cell culture model of syncytin-1 overexpressing cells it has been shown that syncytin-1 is capable of anti-apoptotic functions. A lower apoptotic response, such as a lower level of caspase 3 along with higher amounts of anti-apoptotic Bcl-2 have been found in syncytin-1 transfected cells compared with controls.

In conclusion, the authors propose that fusogenic syncytin-1 may function as an anti-apoptotic glycoprotein during cell-cell fusion processes. Conversely, alterations in the syncytin-1/GCMa system may, in certain circumstances, be followed by placental disturbances and disorders of pregnancy such as pre-eclampsia and IUGR.

In: Human Placenta: Structure and Development... ISBN: 978-1-60876-457-0
Editors: E. Berven, et al. pp. 1-48 © 2010 Nova Science Publishers, Inc.

Chapter I

Human Term Placenta as a Therapeutic Agent: From the First Clinical Applications to Future Perspectives

***Ornella Parolini*[*1], *Abraham Solomon*[2], *Marco Evangelista*[1] *and Maddalena Soncini*[1]**
[1] Centro di Ricerca E. Menni, Fondazione Poliambulanza – Istituto Ospedaliero, Brescia, Italy.
[2] Department of Ophthalmology, Hadassah-Hebrew University Medical Center, Jerusalem, Israel.

Abstract

The placenta is a fetomaternal organ provided by nature to aid development of the growing embryo by facilitating gas and nutrient exchange between the mother and fetus and by helping to maintain fetomaternal tolerance. Aside from playing an age-old and essential role in fetal development, placental tissues have also attracted the interest of clinical scientists due to their potential utility as a therapeutic agent.

For decades, the human term placenta, which is available in plentiful supply and raises no ethical concerns for its procurement, has been used

---

* Corresponding author: Ornella Parolini, Centro di Ricerca E. Menni, Fondazione Poliambulanza – Istituto Ospedaliero, Brescia, Italy, ornella.parolini@tin.it

as a surgical material in skin transplantation, as a biological dressing for treatment of skin wounds, burn injuries and chronic leg ulcers, for prevention of tissue adhesion in surgical procedures, and in ocular surface reconstruction.

More recently, human placenta has also attracted increasing attention from cell and molecular biologists, who have turned to this tissue in the search for a novel stem cell source. Indeed, cells derived from the amniotic and chorionic fetal membranes have been shown to present with high plasticity and to possess low immunogenicity as well as immunomodulatory properties, thereby making them prime candidates for development of cell therapy-based tissue regeneration strategies.

This chapter will provide an overview of the clinical applications which have been described for placental tissue or which are currently applied, and will also give a summary of the most recent results obtained in preclinical studies, which present promising perspectives for the future clinical application of placenta-derived cells.

Amniochorionic Membrane Applications

Fetal membranes, and in particular the amniotic membrane, have been widely used in surgical procedures since the last century. In the earlier literature, amnion and chorion were used interchangeably. In 1910, Davis was the first to report on the use of fetal membranes in skin transplantation [1] by attempting to graft portions of the amniochorionic membrane onto granulating wounds. Shortly after, Sabella and Stern used fetal membranes as a surgical material on burned and ulcerated skin by applying the amniotic membrane directly to the skin surface [2, 3].

Since then, the amniotic and chorionic membranes, either together or separately, have found application in the treatment of open wounds as a temporary biological dressing, in particular in cases of burn injuries, but also for treatment of skin wounds and leg ulcers. Furthermore, some studies have also reported application of the amniochorionic membrane for vaginal reconstruction and orofacial surgery, while experiments in animal models have shown that these tissues are useful for preventing postoperative tissue adhesions in the pelvis and abdomen. However, it is in the field of ophthalmology that the amniotic membrane has found its most extensive utility to date. The use of fetal membranes in this field was introduced in the 1940s by de Rotth, who used both amnion and chorion to replace lost conjunctival tissue [4], while Sorsby later used dried and chemically processed human amniotic membrane as a biological bandage for treating caustic ocular burns [5, 6]. After a period of silence, renewed interest has been ignited in application of the amniotic membrane in ophthalmology, with numerous studies being published in recent years by the group of Tseng and co-workers [7]. Since 2000, several studies have provided further evidence to support the usefulness of the amniotic membrane in ophthalmology, as shown by the extensive available literature which reports applications of this membrane in acute management of chemical burns, conjunctival reconstruction, corneal reconstruction and limbal stem cell deficiency [8-10]. Over the years, different techniques for preservation of the amniotic membrane have been developed, with the final aim of eliminating risk of microbiological and disease transmission generally associated with transplantation of human organs, whilst still retaining the properties of the membrane.

Fetal Membranes as a Surface Covering on Open Wounds

Since the first report by Davis regarding the use of amniochorionic membrane in skin transplantation, this tissue has been applied extensively as a biological dressing on open wounds, forming a good surface covering which has convenient handling properties, and with the added advantages of being thin, adhesive, easy moldable and removable.

Preliminary studies reported by Douglas in 1952, who investigated the amniotic and chorionic membranes as allograft materials for large wounds, in particular those resulting from burns, demonstrate that orientating the membrane so that the mesenchymal layer is in direct contact with the wound results in a more consistent and effective “take”, with neovascularization observed when a chorionic membrane fragment was applied to the burns [11]. Subsequent investigations in sheep by Trelford and colleagues, who used amnion alone as an auto- and allo-graft to cover induced skin defects, confirmed Douglas’s observation regarding the orientation of the membrane [12-14].

During this same period, the usefulness and versatility of human amniochorionic membrane for the treatment of open wounds in a variety of common and challenging clinical situations was demonstrated by several different groups in a large number of patients. These studies showed that treatment with fetal membranes could aid in pain relief, prevention of infections, prevention of heat and fluid loss and promotion of healing. In particular, Robson and colleagues performed studies on 150 patients to investigate the relationship between treatment with fetal membranes and bacterial growth on burn wounds, demonstrating that application of both the amniotic and chorionic layers, instead of the amniotic layer alone, prevents dessication and affords better protection [15-17]. In another study, amniotic membrane alone was used to cover open wounds in rats, and also to dress partial-thickness burns and split-thickness donor sites in 107 patients, and in all cases, no vascularization was detected [18]. Meanwhile, in a cohort study of 120 patients, various clinical types of both traumatic and non traumatic wounds, such as skin ulcers, elective surgical wounds, infected wounds, contaminated surgical wounds, non-healing wounds, burns and traumatic soft-tissue wounds were treated with fetal membranes by applying chorionic membrane to the surface of full-thickness wounds, or applying amniotic membrane to partial–thickness wounds. Depending on the level of the wound, the membranes either served to allow spontaneous closure of the wounds or to prepare the wounds for definitive closure by promoting the growth of healthy granulating tissue [19].

In the years that followed, clinical methods for applying amniotic membrane to treat burns were developed. Indeed, amniochorionic membrane or amniotic membrane alone have both been applied extensively, mainly as skin substitutes for covering burns of different degrees, in particular for partial-thickness burns, as recently reviewed by Kesting [20]. To date, more than 1500 patients with partial-thickness burns are reported to have been treated with amniotic membrane, with reported beneficial effects including promotion of healing and re-epithelialization, pain relief, fluid loss, scar reduction and comfort of dressing changes.

In some cases, comparison between the effects of treatment with amniotic membrane and standard topical treatments or bioengineered skin substitutes, which have the drawbacks of limited viability, limited quantity and high cost, showed that amniotic membrane conferred comparable benefit with respect to these other treatment types [21-27]. For the treatment of partial-thickness burns, fresh amnion has generally been used, while bacterial overgrowth has been controlled through silver nitrate impregnation [21, 22, 26, 28], rinsing with 0.025% sodium hypochlorite solution followed by storage in sterile saline [24, 29], or through gamma irradiation [30, 31]. Cryopreservation by freezing at -80°C [23, 32] or by glycerol preservation at 4°C have also been proposed, with demonstration that tissues stored under these conditions have effects which are comparable with those observed when fresh tissues are used [27, 33].

In some cases, amniotic membrane has also been applied in the management of donor sites for split-thickness skin grafts to cover burns, where less pain and reduced infection was observed after application of saline-preserved amnion on donor regions [34, 35], while on the contrary, severe pain was reported when gamma-irradiated amniotic membrane was used [36].

Treatment of third degree burns with amniotic membrane has been challenging. Even though it has been reported that management of full-thickness burns with amniotic membrane was difficult and frequent infection was noticed [37-39], some subsequent studies have reported the successful use of this tissue in a limited number of patients for treating third degree burns. In this setting, application of the amniotic membrane has been suggested to protect the epithelium when epithelial regeneration has already begun [24]. While use of the amniotic membrane is not recommended on infected wounds, reduced exudation and induration, as well as good re-epithelialization, have all been reported on non-infected wounds treated with this membrane [32]. Finally, treatment of full-thickness burns with microskin grafts covered with fresh amnion has been shown to result in early epithelialization, although it should also be considered that in this study, infections occurred in some cases [40].

Today, the use of amniotic membrane is considered as an accepted and established treatment for partial-thickness burns, especially in developing countries where it is more difficult to find other skin substitutes and where use of amniotic membrane is more practical from an economic point of view [22, 28, 29, 31]. Even recently, the use of amniotic membrane was reported in a clinical trial for the treatment of partial-thickness facial burns in 100 pediatric patients in the USA, with demonstration that this membrane is a safe and effective dressing type compared to standard topical treatments [41].

Application of amniotic membrane to chronic leg ulcers has also been explored. Benefits resulting from this type of treatment for ulcers of different origin were first reported by Gruss [19]. Shortly after, application of amniotic membrane to chronic leg ulcers was shown to promote granulation tissue and vessel formation [42]. When applied to ulcers prior to skin grafting, cultured amniotic membrane promoted a good take of the graft [43]. In a retrospective study of 28 patients, treatment with human amnion prior to split-skin grafting resulted in a 50% ulceration recurrence at 1 year [44]. Interestingly, the beneficial effects conferred by application of amniotic membrane to leg ulcers also seem to be observed when frozen, fresh or lyophilized membrane is used [45].

Even recently, the use of gamma-irradiated amniotic membrane for treating chronic ulcers has been proposed for promoting the closure of non-healing ulcers of different etiologies [46]. Furthermore, in a prospective study on 15 patients, amniotic membrane applied to chronic venous ulcers under a compression bandage was seen to promote epithelialization from the wound edges while suppressing excessive fibrosis. Although promising, it should be noted that when this study was concluded after 3 months, 9 patients still had ulcers [47].

Applications of Amniochorionic Membrane for Vaginoplasty

Some studies have reported the use of amniotic membrane in vaginoplasty for the formation of an artificial vagina or as a graft on the reconstructed organ. The use of amnion for construction of an artificial vagina was first reported by Brindeau and Burger in the 1930s in patients with mullerian agenesis [48, 49], and later by Trelford in patients who had previously undergone anterior exenteration [50]. Furthermore, fragments of unseparated amniochorionic membrane, or of amniotic membrane alone, have both been used to line the artificial constructed vagina in patients with congenital absence of the vagina [51] or in patients undergoing vaginoplasty for various etiologies [52-54], resulting in promotion of re-epithelialisation of the vaginal epithelium. Meanwhile, another study has also reported successful use of amniotic membrane for urethral reconstruction [55].

Applications of Amniochorionic Membrane for Prevention of Postoperative Adhesions

On the basis of a study in which fetal membranes were applied to the pelvises of dogs undergoing pelvic exenteration [56], Trelford went on to report the use of amniotic membrane for replacing the pelvic peritoneum in 12 patients undergoing exenterative procedures, observing an absence of intestinal complications and lack of adhesions [57].

The efficacy of human amniotic membrane in preventing postoperative abdominal and urogenital adhesions was subsequently investigated in animal models.

In particular, amniotic membrane grafts were able to decrease adhesions resulting from bowel perforation, and also to control bacterial contamination in a rabbit model [58]. Meanwhile, application of trypsin-treated, gamma-irradiated human amniotic membrane to injured uterine horns of nulliparous female rabbits resulted in reduced postoperative adhesion: only 4 out of 30 uterine horns treated showed any adhesion formation, while all 24 untreated controls showed adhesion formation [59]. Efficacy in preventing adhesion formation in uterine horns with standard lesions was also shown in a rat model [60].

Viable amniotic membrane has proven to be an excellent anti-adhesive when used in the coverage of peritoneal wall defects in a rat model, with 0-3 % adhesion formation observed 3 weeks after initial surgery in treated animals, compared to control animals which showed 70% adhesion [61]. Furthermore, in a rat model of hernia ventral repair with polypropylene mesh, laying of human amniotic membrane over the abdominal viscera before polypropylene mesh repair resulted in a significant reduction of adhesion formation when compared to treatment with uncovered mesh [62]. Meanwhile, however, failure to prevent adhesion formation has been reported by Badawy et al in a rat model after application of an intra-abdominal amniotic membrane graft [63], as well as in a rabbit model by Arora et al after covering of the uterine horn with gamma-irradiated amniotic membrane [64].

Interestingly, a preclinical study which assessed the usefulness of amniotic membrane as a pericardial substitute in a dog model showed that glutaraldehyde-treated amnion patches were effectively able to serve as biological membranes for pericardial closure, with minimal extrapericardial adhesions and no epicardial adhesion evident 18 weeks after surgery [65].

Moreover, prevention of adhesions has also been reported in animal models when amniotic membrane was applied in combination with hyaluronic acid for tendon repair [66-68].

Applications of Amniochorionic Membrane for Orofacial Defects

In 1985, use of amniotic membrane for the reconstruction of composite orofacial defects was described. In 3 human cases, placement of this membrane over the pectoralis major muscle used for oral cavity reconstruction resulted in more rapid development of the mucosa and less wound contracture compared to controls, suggesting that amniotic membrane enhanced re-epithelialisation of the oral cavity and reduced contracture effects in moderate-sized defects [69]. In human otolaryngology, amniotic membrane has been applied unsuccessfully as a tympanic membrane graft, while good results have been obtained by using this membrane to cover head and neck sites after flap necrosis [70]. The use of amniotic membrane as a biodegradable material for covering the denuded periosteal area after mandibular vestibuloplasty in humans suggests that this membrane may represent a favorable material for promoting healing and preventing relapse [71, 72].

Amniotic Membrane Transplantation in Ophthalmology

Even though the first use of the amniotic membrane in ophthalmology was described by de Rotth in 1940 for the repair of conjunctival defects [4], the amniotic membrane was definitively introduced into ocular surgery almost 15 years ago by the group of Tseng [73] , and its utility has since been described for many applications. A series of experiments in animal models showing amniotic membrane efficacy in various wound healing processes were later followed by numerous clinical reports which have demonstrated a number of applications of this tissue, mostly in ocular surface reconstructive surgery.

The effects of the amniotic membrane are based on 2 basic mechanisms: the ability of the basement membrane of the amniotic membrane to serve as a scaffold for the growth of the ocular surface epithelium in conditions where the epithelium is diseased or absent; and the significant anti-inflammatory and anti-fibrotic effects of the amniotic membrane, which help to suppress the inflammatory and fibrotic processes which are characteristic of most of the severe ocular surface disorders.

Surgical Principles of Amniotic Membrane Transplantation in Ophthalmology

The amniotic membrane can be transplanted onto the ocular surface utilizing one of two major techniques – either as a permanent graft (called the "inlay" technique), where the amniotic membrane is used as a scaffold, over which the adjacent epithelium can grow; or as a temporary biological bandage (also termed the "overlay" technique), where the membrane covers a portion of the ocular surface, and the epithelium is expected to grow underneath the membrane.

The amniotic membrane as a graft (Inlay Technique) - When the amniotic membrane is used as a graft (Figure 1A), it is placed over an area with an epithelial defect or a deep ulcer, with its epithelial side facing up (towards the surgeon) and the stromal side facing the denuded stroma of the ocular surface.

The amniotic membrane is trimmed to fit into the ulcer or defect area, and its basement membrane is used as a scaffold upon which the corneal or the conjunctival epithelium can grow [74] . The membrane can be anchored to the surface with either 10–0 nylon or 10–0 polyglactin sutures, or with fibrin glue [75, 76]. The normal adjacent epithelium is expected to grow over the amniotic membrane, and eventually the amniotic membrane remains and incorporates in the cornea or the conjunctiva as a permanent graft.

A modification of this technique involves "filling in" pieces or multiple layers of the amniotic membrane to build the missing stroma in deep corneal stromal ulcers [77] .

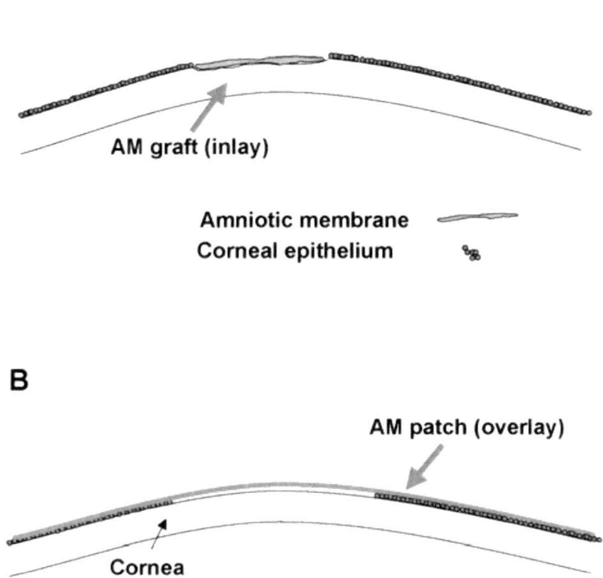

(A) Inlay Technique: the amniotic membrane is used as a permanent graft in persistent epithelial defects of the ocular surface, where it forms a scaffold on which the adjacent epithelium will grow. (B) Overlay Technique: the amniotic membrane is used as a temporary biological bandage, to promote epithelial healing beneath it, and to suppress inflammation. Once epithelial healing is complete, the amniotic membrane dissolves.

Figure 1. Amniotic membrane transplantation techniques in ophthalmology.

The amniotic membrane as a patch (Overlay Technique) - In the overlay technique (Figure 1B), the membrane is used as a temporary biological bandage layer to promote epithelial growth underneath it [78, 79]. The amniotic membrane is placed with its epithelial and basement membrane surface facing either down or upwards. The patch is sutured to the surrounding conjunctiva or episclera with a continuous peri-limbal 10-0 nylon suture, and this may be augmented with multiple interrupted sutures [75]. Fibrin glue can also be used for applying the amniotic membrane. The components of fibrin glue can be applied separately on the amniotic membrane and on the ocular surface. The amniotic membrane with the fibrinogen component is then flipped over the ocular surface into the site of the ulceration, where thrombin has already been applied [80].

Applications of Amniotic Membrane for Acute Management of Chemical Burns

The most important clinical application of the amniotic membrane is as a temporary bandage after acute chemical burns of the ocular surface [81]. The amniotic membrane can be used as an anti-inflammatory patch during acute phases of chemical and thermal burns, whereby it is sutured to cover the entire ocular surface, including the inferior and superior fornices, and acts to limit corneal and limbal inflammation and to reduce symblepharon formation. It is believed that the amniotic membrane may serve as a trap for inflammatory cells that infiltrate the ocular surface after a chemical burn, and that as these cells are caught in the amniotic membrane, they undego apoptosis [82]. In addition, it has been postulated that the amniotic membrane may serve as a collagen substrate for the collagenases that are secreted by inflammatory cells, thereby reducing the ability of these enzymes to digest the corneal stroma collagen. The amniotic membrane may dissolve from a few days to 2 weeks after application, and repeated applications of the amniotic membrane are therefore needed until the ocular surface is completely epithelialized. To address the problem of repeated amniotic membrane applications, a sutureless amniotic membrane device was recently introduced whereby the amniotic membrane layer is anchored on a symblepharon ring, and is applied to the eye in the clinic [83]. In more severe chemical burns (grades III and IV) the amniotic membrane alone may not be enough, and further procedures are needed [84]. Finally, application of amniotic membrane was reported to be sight saving in the management of toxic epidermal necrolysis, preserving normal ocular and eyelid surfaces [85].

Applications of Amniotic Membrane for Conjunctival Reconstruction

The excision of several conjunctival lesions may leave a large defect, which may heal faster if amniotic membrane is transplanted over the defect area.

Pterygium - The efficacy of the amniotic membrane in pterygium surgery, either alone or in conjunction with other modalities, has been established in many reports. When amniotic membrane was used in pterygium surgery in combination with conjunctival or limbal autografts [86], and compared with other methods such as conjunctival autografts [87-89], or with Mitomycin C [87], the amniotic membrane was shown to be as effective as the other methods, and this was especially evident in cases of very large conjunctival defects or primary double-headed pterygium, recurrent pterygia associated with ocular movement restriction and symblephara, or in the context of preserving superior bulbar conjunctiva for future glaucoma surgeries.

However, recent studies have presented controversial results. Studies comparing amniotic membrane transplantation with conjunctival autograft found higher recurrence rates in cases where amniotic membrane was used [90, 91]. It is believed that variations in the surgical procedure and the extent of tissue removal may partially explain this controversy.

Tumors - Amniotic membrane transplantation has been used successfully for reconstruction of both small and large surface defects that result from the excision of conjunctival malignant melanoma, primary acquired melanosis, and other ocular surface squamous neoplasia [92]. In such cases, the use of amniotic membrane bears a number of advantages: its transparency allows monitoring of tumor recurrence and gives a better cosmetic appearance, ocular surface healing occurs rapidly, and tumor recurrence is low. The amniotic membrane replaces other methods such as conjunctival autografts and oral mucous membrane grafts.

Symblepharon Release and Fornix Reconstruction - Amniotic membrane transplantation is effective in fornix reconstruction and symblepharon repair (Figure 2) in a variety of ocular surface disorders, such as ocular cicatricial pemphigoid, after pterygium excision, chemical or mechanical trauma, strabismus surgery, Stevens-Johnson syndrome, toxic epidermal necrolysis, and chronic allergic conjunctivitis [85, 93]. The success rate of fornix reconstruction and repair of symblepharon was 70.6% with the use of amniotic membrane. A recent report found excellent results with intraoperative use of

0.04% Mitomycin C in conjunction with amniotic membrane transplantation for fornix reconstruction in severe cicatricial disease [94].

Other indications - Amniotic membrane transplantation has been shown to be effective for the reconstruction of the conjunctiva after excision of conjunctivochalasis [94]. The amniotic membrane has also been used to manage conjunctival complications after filtering surgery, such as leaking blebs, to cover valve implants, and to cover scleral or pericardial patches [95].

Applications of Amniotic Membrane for Corneal Reconstruction

Corneal Ulcers and Perforations - The management of deep corneal ulcers, corneal and scleral perforations, and persistent epithelial defects is challenging, and often a penetrating keratoplasty or a patch graft is not possible. Amniotic membrane transplants have been used in these cases to fill in the stromal defects and to promote epithelial growth (Figure 3). Several studies have demonstrated the efficacy of multilayered amniotic membrane transplants to manage deep corneal ulcers [77, 96, 97]. In addition, multilayer amniotic membrane was found to be effective in treating corneal perforations smaller than 1.5 mm [98]. Another group used amniotic membrane alone in corneal ulcers and in conjunction with fibrin glue in corneal perforations, in cases such as neurotrophic or exposure ulcers and different autoimmune disorders [99]. This study showed that the use of fibrin glue enhanced the efficacy of the amniotic membrane in sealing corneal perforations of up to 3 mm.

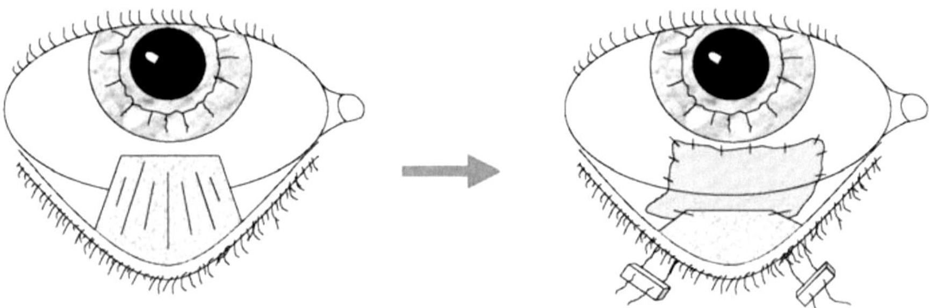

The symblepharon scar tissue (left) is removed, while preserving the epithelium of the symblepharon. A large piece of amniotic membrane is then used to cover the epithelial defect and prevent adhesions and recurrence of the symblepharon.

Figure 2. Symblepharon repair with the amniotic membrane.

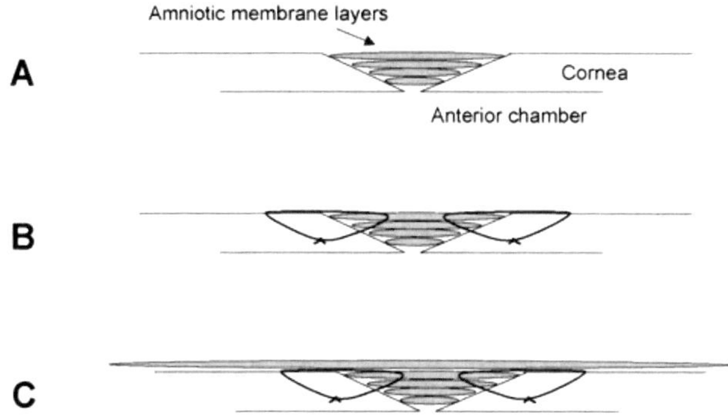

Figure 3. Multiple layers of the amniotic membrane are used to fill in the stromal defect in a deep corneal ulcer.

Persistent Epithelial Defects - Persistent epithelial defects are commonly seen in neurotrophic keratitis, dry eyes, chemical burns, ocular cicatricial pemphigoid, and Stevens-Johnson syndrome. Prolonged inflammation of the ocular surface may damage the limbal epithelial stem cells and the basement membrane. The amniotic membrane may help in these conditions by both suppressing inflammation and promoting epithelial healing. Studies of patients with persistent epithelial defects showed that suturing amniotic membrane grafts in an area corresponding with the epithelial defect helped to promote epithelial healing of these ulcers [78, 100].

Chronic corneal edema (Bullous Keratopathy) - The corneal endothelium is responsible for the regulation of stromal hydration and maintenance of corneal transparency. Damage to the corneal endothelium may be caused by surgical trauma, uncontrolled glaucoma, and Fuchs dystrophy, and usually results in stromal edema and epithelial bullae. Ocular pain with visual loss are seen in these patients.

The amniotic membrane has been used successfully in the treatment of symptomatic bullous keratopathy. The long-term outcomes of epithelial debridement and amniotic membrane transplantation for pain and discomfort relief was demonstrated in patients with symptomatic bullous keratopathy and poor visual potential, whereby pain relief and corneal epithelial healing were obtained in the majority of these patients [101, 102].

Band Keratopathy – Amniotic membrane grafting has also been reported to assist in the management of band keratopathy [103]. Specifically, the amniotic membrane was grafted after surgical removal of calcific deposits with or without the use of ethylenediaminetetraacetic acid (EDTA), resulting in fast corneal epithelialization and resultant surface stability, and resolution of pain in most of the patients.

Applications of Amniotic Membrane in Limbal Stem Cell Deficiency

The amniotic membrane can be used as a substrate for *ex vivo* expansion of either limbal epithelial stem cells or oral mucosal epithelial cells, for subsequent transplantation in cases of total limbal epithelial stem cell deficiency. Limbal epithelial cells from the healthy controlateral eyes of patients with severe unilateral corneal disease can be cultured and expanded on the amniotic membrane. The amniotic membrane, together with the sheet of limbal epithelial cells, is then transplanted onto the denuded corneal surface of the damaged eye after superficial keratectomy to remove fibrovascular ingrowth [104, 105]. Complete re-epithelialization of the corneal surface is evident within a few days of transplantation, with a stable corneal epithelium after long term follow-up.

The same culture system may be used to expand the autologous oral epithelium on the amniotic membrane, which can be subsequently transplanted in cases of bilateral limbal stem cell deficiency [106-108].

Preparation of Amniotic Membrane for Clinical Applications

As for other human tissues or organs, transplantation of amniotic membrane carries a risk of transmission of infectious agents. It is for this reason that today, a detailed social and medical history must be obtained when screening all potential donors. Those who may be at risk of transmitting HIV, HBV or HCV are excluded from donation. Therefore, methods for long-term storage of amniotic membrane, such as cryopreservation or long-term storage in glycerol, are desirable in order to allow checking of donor material, both at the time of procurement and also 6 months afterwards (window period), for HIV 1 and 2, hepatitis B, hepatitis C virus, and syphilis antigens [8, 9]. Infections may also be transmitted during procurement or preparation of the membranes, and aseptic conditions must therefore be maintained at all times during these processes. In this regard, placenta obtained from caesarean sections are preferable, given that those obtained from vaginal deliveries generally seem to show a higher level of contamination than those obtained from caesarean sections [109].

The next challenge is that of achieving correct preservation conditions which ensure maintenance of cell viability and other properties of the amniotic membrane which are paramount to its clinical utility.

In the history of clinical application of fetal membranes, various methods for their sterilization and preparation have been proposed. Fresh membranes have often been used, while storage at temperatures above 0°C has also been employed, which allows maintenance of cell viability, although this has been seen to decrease after extended storage periods.

In the first studies to assess methods for amniotic membrane storage, placing of the membrane in saline solution with a mixture of antibiotics (polymixin, ampicillin, gentamicin, amphotericin B) was shown to maintain sterility for at least 48 hours [50, 57]. Meanwhile, membranes which were rinsed in a 0.025% sodium hypochlorite solution before being placed in a sterile saline solution at 4°C could be stored for up to 6 weeks whilst maintaining cell viability and sterility [17, 19] . Later, Haberal et al. proposed that membranes could be soaked in 0.5% silver nitrate for at least 2 hours in order to improve their manageability and antibacterial effects [21]. Interestingly, silver nitrate impregnation was recently reintroduced to increase the antimicrobial properties of amniotic membrane, through deposition of silver by in situ reduction onto the membrane, [28].

Other methods for membrane storage include freeze-drying (lyophilization) or air-drying, followed by gamma irradiation. The freeze-drying method was introduced by Tseng in 1998, and has been well-described by Gajiwala. Specifically, after treatment with 70% ethanol, the amniotic membrane is freeze-dried under a vacuum in order to remove 95% of its moisture [30]. Meanwhile, air-drying is performed by simply placing the membrane in a laminar flow cabinet [31, 39]. In both cases, the packed and sealed amniotic membranes are then sterilized by exposure to 25 kGy radiation, which has been shown to be a suitable method for sterilization of tissue allografts [31, 46]. Air dried, gamma irradiated amniotic membranes have been used efficiently on burns, and have been shown to favour second-degree burn wound healing with no significant differences in clinical efficacy compared to glycerol-preserved amniotic membrane [31].

Among the possible methods for long-term storage, cryopreservation of the amniotic membrane is currently the most widely employed, especially for applications in ophthalmology, and is usually performed by following one of two different protocols. By the first method, proposed by the group of Tseng, the amniochorionic membrane is washed in antibiotic saline solution and the amnion is then separated from the chorion, flattened onto nitrocellulose paper with its epithelial surface facing upwards, and cut into pieces. The membrane fragments are then placed in a sterile vial containing 50% glycerol in Dulbecco's modifies Eagle medium and frozen at –80°C. Immediately before use, the membrane fragments are thawed and rinsed in normal buffered saline at room temperature [7]. The second method, proposed by the group of Tsubota, involves washing of the amniochorionic membrane in physiological saline, before cutting it into pieces and rinsing in PBS. After 3 consecutive 5-minute rinses in PBS containing increasing DMSO concentrations (0.5 M, 1.0 M and 1.5 M), the membrane is placed in a plastic container and frozen at –80°C. At the time of use, the amniochorionic membrane is warmed to room temperature and rinsed in saline, and the amniotic membrane is then separated from the chorion [8, 110]. Cryopreservation allows fetal membranes to retain their properties, even though cell viability has been observed to be greatly reduced or even completely lost after thawing. Interestingly, however, Hennerbichler and colleagues recently reported a cell viability of 13%-18% after freezing of the amniotic membrane for 3 weeks [111]. Further work is therefore warranted to identify the optimal cryopreservation conditions for the amniotic membrane that would give maximal cell viability upon thawing.

Long-term preservation of amniotic membrane in 85% glycerol at 4°C has been most often applied when the membrane is to be used for the treatment of burns. This method was first proposed by Maral for the treatment of partial thickness burns in rats, showing that the membrane remains structurally intact during the preservation process, and that membranes stored under these conditions can be as effective as fresh amnion for the treatment of burns. By this technique, the amniotic membrane is rinsed and separated from the chorion before being placed in 85% glycerol at room temperature for 24 hours. It is then transferred into fresh 85% glycerol and stored at 4°C [27, 33]. This very simple method results in preservation of cell integrity [33] and allows storage of the membrane for up to 2.5 years [27, 33], although cell viability is largely lost [111]. Immediately prior to use, the amniotic membrane fragments need to be rehydrated through immersion in phosphate buffered saline solution for at least 10 minutes.

Clearly, long term storage methods which ensure preservation of cell integrity, as well as methods for preventing transmission of infectious agents, both represent hurdles which need to be overcome in the management and handling of placenta-derived materials. However, depending on the clinical application, retention of cell viability may not always be necessary, and in addition, even though there are numerous studies reporting the low immunogenicity and immunomodulatory properties of amniotic membrane-derived cells, caution should still be exercised considering the possibility that viable allogeneic amniotic cells may be rejected. Although much work remains to be done in this regard, growing interest in the clinical applicability of placental cells and tissues strongly warrants the undertaking of such studies in order to allow routine use of these materials to become a clinical reality.

Applications of Placenta-Derived Cells

In recent years, much interest has been turned toward the placenta in the search for new sources of stem cells. The hypothesis that placental tissues may harbour progenitor cells is supported by the fact that these tissues originate very early during embryogenesis, prior to gastrulation, thereby suggesting that cells from these tissues may retain some of the plasticity that is characteristic of pre-gastrular embryonic cells. Furthermore, the low immunogenicity and the immunomodulatory properties displayed by cells derived from placental tissues suggest that they may be applicable in an allo-transplantation setting and would have a low risk of inducing immunological rejection after transplantation, as already demonstrated clearly by the pre-clinical and clinical studies described above in which the amniotic membrane has been applied in toto.

In recent years, cells derived from the placenta, and in particular from the amniotic and chorionic fetal membranes, have been investigated by several groups who have shown that they display stem cell characteristics, as recently reviewed by Parolini (Figure 4) [112, 113].

The therapeutic potential of placenta-derived cells has also been explored by evaluating their engraftment potential and their regenerative and tissue repair capacity in preclinical studies using several different animal models. As a result of such studies, the list of potential clinical applications of fetal membrane-derived cells is growing continuously.

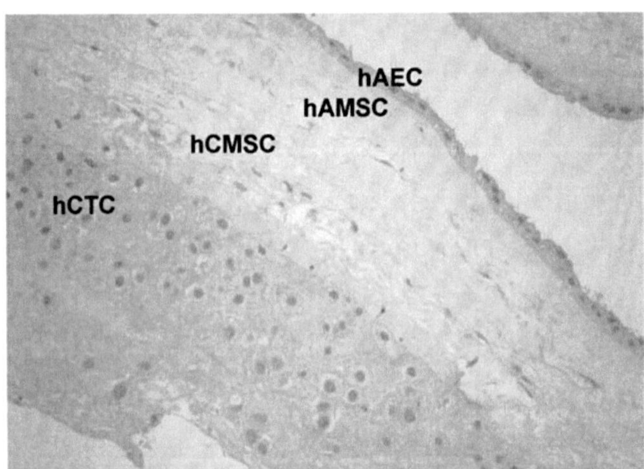

Fetal membrane section stained with hematoxilin-eosin. hAEC: human amniotic epithelial cells; hAMSC: human amniotic mesenchymal stromal cells; hCMSC: human chorionic mesenchymal stromal cells; hCTC: human chorionic trophoblastic cells.

Figure 4. Human fetal membrane-derived cells.

Engraftment of Placenta-derived Cells in Allogeneic and Xenogeneic Animal Models

In the previous paragraphs, we have seen that the amniotic membrane in toto has been widely used as a therapeutic agent in different procedures without causing any signs of rejection. Furthermore, it has also been shown that cells isolated from placental tissues and injected as suspensions into immunocompetent animal models are able to engraft long term without signs of immunological rejection. This indicates active tolerance of the transplanted cells, which is a key feature that would be essential to permit their use in different clinical applications.

Indeed, prolonged survival of human amnion-derived cells has been demonstrated by various groups after xenogeneic transplantation into organs of various animal models, including survival for at least 60 days in the injured spinal cord of bonnet monkeys [114], for 2 months in infarcted rat myocardium [115], for 5 weeks in the injured spinal cord of rats [116], for 4 weeks in the injured striatum of mice [117], and for 3 weeks in the ischemic rat brain [118]. Meanwhile, long-term engraftment up to 120 days after transplantation, as well as migration into different organs, have been observed after intravenous transplantation of human amniochorionic cells into newborn swine and rats, with human microchimerism detected in the bone marrow, brain, lung and thymus of these animals, thereby suggesting active migration and integration into specific organs, as well as active tolerance of the xenogeneic cells [119].

After allogeneic in utero transplantation of rat amnion-derived cells into the developing rodent brain at embryonic day 15.5, long-term survival for up to two and half months postnatally has also been described in different regions of the brain of recipient animals, with no evidence of immunological rejection [120].

Finally, human placenta-derived mesenchymal stem cells labelled with bisbenzimide and injected into the peritoneum of fetal rats in utero have been shown to engraft in 60% of the recipients with no evidence of rejection. Even though the majority of the transplanted cells were seen to migrate to the placenta, some cells were also detectable in fetal organs including the brain, lung, heart, liver and spleen, and these cells persisted in the recipient animals for at least 12 weeks after birth. Very interestingly, immunostaining of serial sections of the engrafted organs of these animals with lineage-specific markers led the authors to hypothesize that the cells had undergone specific differentiation after transplantation [121].

The *in vivo* migratory capabilities of placenta-derived cells which are evident from some of the experiments above have been ascribed to the expression of surface adhesion and migratory molecules including integrins, CD54 (ICAM-1), E-cadherin, CD50 (ICAM-3), CD56 (NCAM), CD102 (ICAM –2), CD106 (VCAM-1), VLA (very late antigen) –5, and the matrix receptors CD44 and CD166 (ALCAM) [119, 122]. Furthermore, intracellular chemokine receptor protein expression has also been detected in placenta derived cells, which may further aid the migration of these cells *in vivo* [122].

Placenta-derived Cells for Regenerating Neural Functions

The majority of the preclinical studies which have been performed using placenta-derived cells describe transplantation of amniotic epithelial cells into animal models with neurological injuries. Such experiments have been undertaken on the basis of *in vitro* studies which suggest that these cells may have a predisposition toward the neural lineage. In particular, amniotic epithelial cells have been reported to express neural lineage markers including nestin, MAP2 and GFAP [123-125], as well as performing neuronal functions including synthesis and release of acetylcholine, catecholamines and neurotrophic factors [126-131]. Finally, these cells have also been shown to be capable of supporting *in vitro* growth of neural cell types [129, 132-134]. Further support to the hypothesized neural predisposition of placenta-derived cells comes from studies which demonstrate positivity for the neural progenitor marker nestin and the mature neuron marker NF200 not only for amniotic membrane-derived cells, but also for chorion- and trophoblast villous- derived cells after *in vitro* culture in neurogenic medium [135].

Preclinical studies which have been performed in animal models of brain ischemia, Parkinson's disease and spinal cord injury, even though usually undertaken in limited numbers of animals, nevertheless suggest that amniotic cells of either human or animal origin are able to confer neuroprotective and neuroregenerative effects, as recently reviewed by Yu and collegues [136].

In particular, several studies have indicated the potential of amniotic epithelial cells for restoring neural function in cerebral ischemia. For example, Okawa and colleagues have demonstrated that when transplanted into the ischemic brain of immunocompetent adult gerbils, rat amniotic epithelial cells which were cultured for 4 days and then labelled with the fluorescent dye PKH26, were able to survive for at least 5 weeks, migrating into the pyramidal layer and retaining positivity for the neuronal marker MAP2 [125]. Meanwhile, Liu and colleagues have shown that after transplantation of human amniotic epithelial cells into the striatum of ischemic rats, these cells were able to survive for 3 weeks and express the neural lineage markers MAP2, nestin and GFAP, while amelioration of behavioural dysfunction in coordination and motor tests, and reduction in the size of infarcted areas in cell-treated animals compared to controls, was also observed. These effects were more evident when the amniotic epithelial cells were transduced with the glial cell line-derived neurotrophic factor (GDNF), as compared to cells which had been transduced with enhanced green fluorescent protein (EGFP) [118].

Furthermore, in two different animal models of Parkinson's disease, human amniotic epithelial cells labelled with PKH26 and implanted into the brain have been shown to confer beneficial effects. In particular, in a rat model of Parkinson's disease induced by intrastriatal infusions of 6-hydroxydopamine, transplantation of human amniotic epithelial cells into the midbrain of immunosuppressed animals resulted in dopamine production, prevention of nigral dopamine neuron degeneration and in improved performance in a locomotor test for at least 2-4 weeks [137, 138]. The neuroprotective effects of amniotic epithelial cells in Parkinson's disease is further supported by a recent study in which endogenous neurogenesis and behavioural improvement was observed for 4 weeks after transplantation of human amniotic epithelial cells into the striatum of a mouse model of MPTP-induced Parkinson's disease [117].

Beneficial effects of amniotic epithelial cells have also been reported for spinal cord injury repair. In a study by Sankar and colleagues, human amniotic epithelial cells were labelled with the fluorescent dye Dil after 2 days of culturing and were then transplanted into lesioned areas of 4 bonnet monkeys which served as a contusion model of spinal cord injury. The transplanted cells were shown to survive for up to 60 days, and also supported the growth of host axons, enhanced survival of axotomized spinal cord neurons and improved performance in locomotor tests [114]. Moreover, in another study by Meng and colleagues, co-injection of bFGF-expressing rat amniotic epithelial cells and neural stem cells into the brains of spinal cord-injured rats was shown to result in enhanced survival and neural differentiation of both the injected neural stem cells and also host neurons, as well as in significant locomotor improvement for the duration of the study (5 weeks) [116].

Finally, in a study investigating the potential of amniotic epithelial cells to treat a monkey model of the lysosomal storage disorder mucopolisaccharidosis type VII, which causes pathological brain abnormalities, survival and distribution of intra-cerebrally injected monkey amniotic epithelial cells was observed in different regions of the brains of transplanted animals for 1 month [139].

Placenta-derived Cells for Regenerating Cardiomyogenic/Angiogenic Functions

To date, only a few studies have reported on the use of mesenchymal stromal cells from amnion and chorion for improvement of impaired cardiac function in animal models.

The first evidence of the cardiomyogenic potential of human amniotic mesenchymal stromal cells comes from a study which reports that these cells basally express cardiac-specific genes including the cardiac-specific transcription factor GATA4, atrial myosin light chain *(MLC)-2a*, ventricular *MLC-2v* and the cardiac troponins *cTnI* and *cTnT*. In this same study, after labelling of the cells with PKH26 and transplantation into rat hearts following myocardial infarction, the cells were shown to survive for at least 2 months and engraft into cardiac tissue. Furthermore, the transplanted cells were also shown to differentiate into cardiomyocyte-like cells, as demonstrated by immunohistochemical positivity for the cardiac-specific proteins atrial natriuretic peptide (ANP) and β–myosin heavy chain (β-MHC) [115]. In another study, cardiomyocytic differentiation potential was reported for human amniotic epithelial cells after culture of these cells in cardiomyocytic induction medium. After culture, expression of the precursor marker GATA4 and of the differentiated cell markers ANP, MYL7 (myosin light chain 7), CACNA1C (calcium channel, voltage-dependant, L type, α 1C subunit) and KCND3 (potassium voltage-gated channel, Shal-related subfamily member 3) was detected [140].

Beneficial effects of transplanting human amniochorionic-derived cells into infarcted rat hearts have also been reported by Ventura and colleagues, who observed increased capillary density at the infarct border zone, normalization of left ventricular function and significant decreases in scar tissue 4 weeks after the transplant procedure. Interestingly, enhancement of the cardiac differentiation of these cells was observed after treatment of the cells with a mixed ester of hyaluronan and butyric and retinoic acids (HBR), which resulted in increased expression of cardiomyogenic genes (GATA4 and NKX.2) and cardiac proteins (sarcomeric myosin heavy chain and alfa sarcomeric actin) [141]. Furthermore, exposure of the cells to HBR also appeared to enhance cardiovascular repair in infarcted rat hearts after transplantation [141].

Cardiomyogenic potential has also been reported for freshly isolated cells of the chorionic plate, which have been shown to express human cardiomyocyte specific-genes such as genes of cardiac transcription factors Csx/Nkx-2.5 and GATA4, brain natriuretic peptide (BNP), cTnT, cardiac actin and MLC-2a. Meanwhile, co-culture of these cells after 5 to 9 passages with murine fetal cardiomyocytes, which served to induce cardiac differentiation, resulted in spontaneous beating of the chorionic cells starting from day 3 and continuing until day 21 after the beginning of co-culture [142].

In addition to the cardiac-specific features which have been described for placenta-derived cells, angiogenic potential of these cells has also been reported in *in vitro* studies. In particular, amniotic membrane-derived cells have been shown to basally express the endothelial specific markers FLT-1 and KDR, and are able to spontaneously organize into capillary-like structures when cultured on semisolid medium. Expression of endothelial markers by these cells seems to increase after exposure to HBR or VEGF [141, 143].

Finally, endothelial differentiation of placenta-derived cells has also been suggested by the study of Wu and colleagues, who cultured placenta-derived multipotent cells obtained from the trophoblast in media containing endothelial growth factors for 3 days, together with application of physiological levels of shear stress for 24 hours. Under these conditions, increased expression of vWF (von Willebrand Factor) and PECAM-1 (platelet-endothelial cell adhesion molecule-1) at both the gene and protein levels, as well as formation of tube-like structures, were observed by 3 hours after exposure to shear stress, and were sustained over the entire 24-hour period [144].

Placenta-derived Cells for Regenerating Hepatic Function

The first attempt to investigate whether human amniotic epithelial cells can perform hepatic functions *in vivo* is documented in the study of Sakuragawa and coworkers, who reported that some of these cells can express albumin and α-fetoprotein. In addition, after transplantation of human amniotic epithelial cells which had been transduced with the β-galactosidase gene into the livers of SCID mice, integration of transplanted α-fetoprotein- and albumin-positive cells was observed in the hepatic parenchyma at 1 and 2 weeks after cell injection. From these observations, the authors suggest that human amniotic epithelial cells could prove useful as transgene carriers for allogeneic cell transplantation into the liver [145]. Later studies have investigated the hepatocytic differentiation potential of human amniotic epithelial cells, showing that when cultured in hepatocytic induction medium, these cells express liver-specific transcription factors including hepatocyte nuclear factor (HNF)-3γ and HNF-4α, CCAAT/enhancer-binding protein (CEBP)- α and -β and CYP450 enzymes [146, 147]. Meanwhile, hepatic functions such as albumin production at heterogeneous levels and glycogen storage have also been shown for human amniotic epithelial cells [140, 145, 146].

Further evidence that amniotic tissues may perform hepatocyte-related functions comes from a study showing that implantation of human amniotic membrane into the peritoneum of SCID mice resulted in detection of human albumin in sera and peritoneal fluid of the transplanted animals from day 1 to day 7 (duration of the study) [146].

Interestingly, amniotic membrane in toto as well as amniotic epithelial cells have also been proposed for the treatment of the Niemann-Pick disease, a lysosomal storage disorder which is caused by a deficiency in the activity of sphingomyelinase, resulting in hepatosplenomegaly and accumulation of sphingomyelin in different organs. In a study by Scaggiante and colleagues, six subcutaneous implantations of minced human amniotic membrane were performed at intervals of 1-4 months into the thoracic pouch under the armpit of a young patient, resulting in successful enzyme replacement as demonstrated by improvement in the patient's clinical condition (intestinal absorption, body weight, decrease of hepatomegaly) [148]. Furthermore, *in vitro* experiments have indicated that human amniotic epithelial cells can spontaneously secrete considerable amounts of some lysosomal enzymes [149], and repeated implantation of these cells, which served as a source of exogenous sphingomyelinase, has been shown to lead to improvements in the general conditions of five young patients. In particular, in two of these cases, a single implantation caused a sustained normalization of sphingomyelin and total phospholipids in urine [150]. Even though very preliminary, these data nevertheless indicate the potential of amniotic membrane-derived cells for use in the treatment of a broad spectrum of metabolic diseases.

Placenta-derived Cells for Regenerating Pancreatic Function

Pancreatic functions of amniotic epithelial cells have also been observed by some groups. Wei et al. reported correction of hyperglycemia for at least 1 month in streptozotocin-induced diabetic SCID mice which had undergone intrasplenic transplantation of insulin-producing human amniotic epithelial cells that had first been cultured in the presence of nicotinamide for 2-4 weeks [151]. Similar findings were reported by Chang and colleagues, who cultured placenta-derived multipotent stem cells in a pancreatic induction medium for 4 weeks, and subsequently observed formation of 3D spheroid bodies expressing mature pancreas-related genes such as insulin, glucagon (also observed at the protein level) and somatostatin. Furthermore, transplantation of the spheroid bodies into the left kidneys of streptozotocin-pretreated SCID mice, a site which is known to provide a microenvironment that stimulates endocrine cell differentiation, resulted in implantation of insulin- and glucagon- positive cells and in restoration of normoglycemia until 4 weeks after transplantation [152]. The pancreatic differentiation potential of human amniotic epithelial cells was further confirmed in another study whereby these cells were cultured in pancreatic induction media, resulting in the display of ultrastructural features characteristics of β- pancreatic cells, as well as expression of the pancreatic exocrine cell marker AMY2B (amylase α2B) and production of glucagon [140].

Placenta-derived Cells for Treatment of Pulmonary Fibrosis

Very recently, the effects of fetal membrane-derived cells on lung fibrosis were investigated in a large study which included 197 animals. Pulmonary fibrosis was induced in mice by intra-tracheal instillation of bleomycin , followed by either intra-tracheal, intra-peritoneal or intra-venous injection of allogeneic (mouse into mouse) or xenogeneic (human into mouse) amniochorionic cells. Reduced levels of bleomycin-induced lung fibrosis were subsequently observed, as demonstrated by reductions in fibroblast infiltration and collagen deposition (Figure 5), and interestingly, these beneficial effects were seen independently of the cell delivery route or donor cell source (allo- or xenogeneic) [153].

Properties and Effects of Amniotic Membrane

Immunomodulatory Properties of Amnion

For many years, immunologists have been intrigued by the placenta due to the fact that this organ contributes to maintenance of fetomaternal tolerance and very likely harbours the fundamental mechanisms of immunological tolerance. Several mechanisms have been proposed to explain maternal acceptance of the fetus: from the Medawar hypothesis [154] to other site-specific immunosuppressive mechanisms such as expression of non-classical MHC molecules, or expression of the IDO enzyme, FasL, or complement regulator proteins by placental cells (reviewed by [155-157]).

The fact that placental tissues contribute to fetomaternal tolerance suggests that cells present within these tissues may be immune-privileged, thereby making them an ideal tool for therapeutic application.

Since the beginning of the 20th century, several clinical studies, such as those discussed previously, have shown that the amniochorionic membrane can be applied for the treatment of open wounds, for the prevention of postoperative tissue adhesions, and in surgical procedures for ocular surface reconstruction, all without rejection in the absence of immunosuppressive treatment (as revised by Trelford [158]).

Furthermore, *in vivo* studies in animal models have reported prolonged survival of fetal membrane-derived cells after xenogeneic transplantation into immunocompetent animals including rats [115-119], swine [119] and bonnet monkeys [114], again with no evidence of immunological rejection. Long term cell survival has also been observed after allogeneic transplantation of rat amnion-derived cells into the rodent brain [120].

Low immunogenicity of fetal membranes has been attributed to low expression of classical MHC class I and II antigens [159, 160].

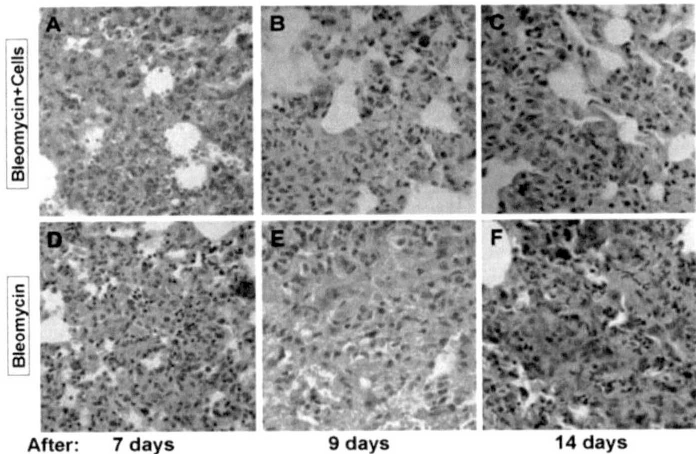

Lung histological sections stained with Masson's trichrome (magnification 40X) to show collagen deposition. (D-E-F) Control samples from non transplanted bleomycin-treated mice collected 7,9 and14 days after intratracheal bleomycin instillation (4U/kg). (A-B-C) Lungs from bleomycin-treated mice collected 7, 9 and 14 days after intra-peritoneal injection (xeno-IP) of xenogeneic fetal membrane-derived cells.

Figure 5. Transplantation of placenta-derived cells decreases bleomycin-induced lung fibrosis in a mouse model.

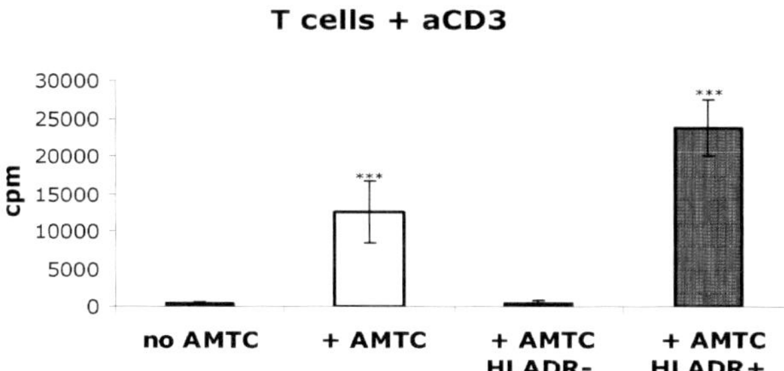

Purified T cells in the presence of anti-CD3 were cultured alone or in direct contact with total amniotic mesenchymal tissue cells (AMTC), HLA-DR-negative AMTC or HLA-DR-positive AMTC. T-cell proliferation was then assessed by [3H]-thymidine incorporation after 3 days of culture and expressed in cpm. Data are mean and SD from at least four independent experiments. , *p* .001 versus corresponding control sample.

Figure 6. Stimulatory effect of HLA-DR-positive cells of the amniotic mesenchymal region on CD3-stimulated T cells.

In vitro studies aimed at understanding the mechanisms underlying the immunological features of fetal membrane-derived cells have shown that these cells do not induce an allogeneic or xenogeneic immune response in a mixed lymphocyte reaction (MLR), and actively suppress T-cell proliferation which has been induced either by an allogeneic stimulus in MLR or by stimulation through the TCR receptor [119, 161-163]. Suppression of T cell proliferation was shown to be maintained in a study where amnion-derived cells were immortalized by ectopic expression of the catalytic subunit of human telomerase (hTERT) which resulted in elongated life span [164].

Recently, it has been shown that amniotic membrane-derived cells are not only capable of eliciting inhibitory effects on T cell proliferation, but also stimulatory effects, as demonstrated by a study in which a stimulatory cell subpopulation with monocyte-macrophage characteristics (positive for HLA-DR, CD45, CD14 and CD11b) was isolated from within the human amniotic mesenchymal region (Figure 6) [162].

Furthermore, the immunomodulatory effects exterted by amniotic membrane-derived cells seem not only to be directed at T cells, but also antigen presenting cells. Indeed, *in vitro* studies have shown that amniotic membrane-derived cells are able to inhibit maturation of monocytes into dendritic cells, preventing the expression of the dendritic cell marker CD1a and reducing the expression of HLA-DR, CD80 and CD83. This blocking of monocyte maturation was associated with an impairment in the allostimulatory ability of these cells on allogeneic T cells [165].

Anti-inflammatory Properties of Amnion

The amniotic membrane has been shown to possess anti-inflammatory and anti-fibrotic properties in several clinical studies centred on surgical reconstruction of the ocular surface [7, 73, 110, 166, 167], as well as in *in vitro* models [168-170].

Several studies have also been performed to investigate the regulation of cytokines associated with inflammatory and fibrotic responses by amniotic membrane-derived cells. In particular, mRNAs of the anti-inflammatory cytokines IL-1ra (receptor antagonist) and IL-10 have been detected in both epithelial and mesenchymal amniotic cells [171]. Similarly, expression of IL-1ra has been shown to be upregulated after culture of corneal limbal epithelial cells on the stromal matrix of human amniotic membrane [172]. Moreover, conditioned medium from human amniotic epithelial cells harvested after 2 days of culture has been shown to suppress inflammation in a murine corneal inflammation model. However, the low concentration of IL-ra detected in the conditioned medium resulted to be only slightly effective in suppression of corneal inflammation, suggesting that other soluble factors may be responsible of the anti-inflammatory effects of amniotic epithelial cells [173].

In an *in vitro* model of allergic stimulation by mast cells and eosinophils, Solomon and colleagues have shown that anti-inflammatory effects exerted by amniotic membrane-derived cells may be partially mediated through down-regulation of production of TGF-β1 (the major fibrogenic cytokine), GM-CSF and IL-8 (cytokines that participate in allergic inflammation responses) by fibroblasts [170].

Meanwhile, a recent *in vitro* study by Magatti and colleagues showed that production of the inflammatory cytokines TNF-α, CXCL10, CXCL9 and CCL5 by mature dendritic cells was inhibited when dendritic cell maturation was induced in the presence of amniotic membrane-derived cells [165].

It has also been hypothesised that the anti-inflammatory actions exerted by the amniotic membrane are mediated by inducing apoptosis of macrophages, which play a key role in initiating, maintaining and resolving host inflammatory responses. Indeed, apoptotic monocytes and macrophages have been found in the matrix of the amniotic membrane 1 week after being placed as a temporary graft on the ocular surface of patients with persistent corneal epithelial defects, suggesting that the amniotic membrane attracts and traps inflammatory cells infiltrating the ocular surface [169]. Furthermore, *in vitro* studies have shown that interferon-γ-activated mouse macrophages underwent increased apoptosis when cultured on amniotic membrane, and this phenomenon seems to be related to downregulation by the amniotic membrane of anti-apoptotic NF-κB and Akt-FKHR signalling pathways [174].

Antiangiogenic Effects of Amnion

Even though early studies in which amniotic membrane was applied to leg ulcers prior to skin grafting reported induction of vessel proliferation [42, 43], later studies reported antiangiogenic effects when amniotic membrane was applied to the corneal surface of ophthalmological patients [73], where neovascularization is a common pathological condition resulting from inflammation [175].

It has been reported that mRNA for antiangiogenic proteins, such as tissue inhibitors of metalloproteinases (TIMP-1, -2, -3, -4), thrombospondin-1 (TSP-1) and collagen XVIII (precursor protein of endostatin) are expressed by amniotic epithelial and mesenchymal cells in glycerol-cryopreserved amniotic membrane [171].

Moreover corneal neovascularization induced by bFGF in a rabbit model has been shown to be significantly reduced by human amniotic membrane conditioned medium. This effect was explained by *in vitro* studies which showed inhibition of vascular endothelial cell migration and cell growth when these cells were cultured in the presence of amniotic cell conditioned medium [176].

In another study, the potent antiangiogenic factor PEDF (pigment epithelium-derived factor) was found to be highly enriched in the basal membrane of human amnion. In particular, the viability of endothelial cells was shown to be decreased in the presence of soluble proteins extracted from the amniotic membrane, and this effect seemed to be partially neutralized by a specific anti-PEDF antibody [177].

Recently, amniotic membrane extract which had been boiled for 30 minutes was shown to inhibit neovessel growth in an alkali-burned corneal neovascularization rat model when applied immediately after injury. *In vitro* studies demonstrated that this effect may be due to inhibition of both endothelial cell proliferation and tube formation. However, expression of PEDF was not detected in the boiled amniotic membrane extract, suggesting that other soluble factors may have been responsible for the inhibitory effects observed [178].

Promotion of Epithelialization by Amnion

Amniotic membrane has been shown to promote epithelialization when applied in different clinical scenarios, and several growth factors produced by this membrane appear to be involved in this process, including epithelial growth factor (EGF), keratinocyte growth factor (KGF), hepatocyte growth factor (HGF), basic fibroblast growth factor (bFGF), transforming growth factor- α (TGF-α), TGF-β [166, 179]. In particular, these factors are expressed predominantly in the epithelial layer of the amnion and can be detected at both the mRNA and protein level, and are still present in cryopreserved amniotic membrane 1 month after the freezing [179].

Anti-microbial Properties of Amnion

The anti-microbial activity of the amniotic membrane was first explored in studies by Robson and colleagues who observed a significant decrease in bacterial counts when rat wounds inoculated with *Pseudomonas aeruginosa* were covered with human amniochorionic membrane as compared to those which had been covered with skin grafts [16]. In a second infection experiment on skin defects created on the backs of rats, amniochorionic membrane resulted equal to autografts in decreasing bacterial counts, but superior to allografted and xenografted skin [17].

More recently, both the amniotic and chorionic membranes have proven effective in inhibiting growth of a wide range of bacteria, including *Hemolytic streptococcus group A*, *Staphylococcus aureus*, *Escherichia Coli* and *Pseudomonas aeruginosa* [180].

While several antimicrobial factors, such as lysozyme [181, 182], transferrin [182] and lactoferrin [183] have been detected in amniotic fluid, these have not been detected in amniochorionic membrane. Talmi and colleagues argue that the dominant mechanism responsible for the antibacterial activity of these membranes is their close adherence to the wound, as demonstrated by complete inhibition of the growth of five types of bacterial under discs of amniotic or amniochorionic membrane or other synthetic membranes [184]. This theory was later confirmed by Kjaergaard who demonstrated that amniotic membrane constitutes an effective physical barrier against infection by group B streptococcus [185].

Conclusion

Sourced from nature itself, the human term placenta represents a tissue which shows great therapeutic potential. Interest in the placenta dates back to the time of Leonardo, who in his anatomy handbooks wrote "*The child in the uterus has three membranes which surround it. Of these, the first is called the amnion, the second the allantois, the third the secundine (chorion). The uterus is united to its secundine by means of the cotyledons, and all join in the umbilical cord which is composed of vessels*" (translated from "Quaderni di Anatomia", folio19v by Leonardo da Vinci). Since the time of Leonardo, it is probable that placental tissues have been applied therapeutically in a myriad of different clinical situations.

Even though the first scientific reports describing clinical application of placental tissues began to emerge one century ago, scientists today continue to investigate which methods may be best for applying the placenta in different clinical settings, with particular focus on characterization of the different cell types present in placental tissues. Indeed, studies now suggest that placenta-derived cells may be useful for repairing damaged or diseased tissues by substituting cells or by secreting factors which modulate the surrounding host environment into which they have been transplanted. In advancing on the findings which have been reported to date, the main goal of research in this area for the coming years will be that of demonstrating *in vivo* differentiation of placenta-derived cells.

References

[1] Davis, J. (1910) Skin transplantation with a review of 550 cases at The Johns Hopkins Hospital. *Johns Hopkins Med J, 15*, 307.

[2] Sabella, N. (1913) Use of the fetal membranes in skin grafting. *Med Rec N Y, 83*, 478.

[3] Stern, M. (1913) The grafting of preserved amniotic membrane to burned and ulcerated surfaces, substituting skin grafts. *JAMA, 60*, 973.

[4] de Rotth, A. (1940) Plastic repair of conjunctival defects with fetal membranes. *Arch Ophthalmol 23*, 522-525.

[5] Sorsby, A. & Symons, H. M. (1946) AMNIOTIC MEMBRANE GRAFTS IN CAUSTIC BURNS OF THE EYE: (Burns of the second degree). *Br J Ophthalmol, 30*, 337-45.

[6] Sorsby, A., Haythorne, J. & Reed, H. (1947) Further Experience with Amniotic Membrane Grafts in Caustic Burns of the Eye. *Br J Ophthalmol, 31*, 409-18.

[7] Tseng, S. C., Prabhasawat, P. & Lee, S. H. (1997) Amniotic membrane transplantation for conjunctival surface reconstruction. *Am J Ophthalmol, 124*, 765-74.

[8] Dua, H. S. & Azuara-Blanco, A. (1999) Amniotic membrane transplantation. *Br J Ophthalmol, 83*, 748-52.

[9] Dua, H. S., Gomes, J. A., King, A. J. & Maharajan, V. S. (2004) The amniotic membrane in ophthalmology. *Surv Ophthalmol, 49*, 51-77.

[10] John, T. (2003) Human amniotic membrane transplantation: past, present, and future. *Ophthalmol Clin North Am, 16*, 43-65, vi.

[11] Douglas, B. (1952) Homografts of fetal membranes as a covering for large wounds; especially those from burns; an experimental and clinical study. *J Tn State Med Assoc, 45*, 230-5.

[12] Trelford, J. D., Anderson, D. G., Hanson, F. W., Mendel, V. & Sawyer, R. H. (1972) Considerations of the amnion as an autograft and as an allograft in sheep. A preliminary report. *J Med, 3*, 231-41.

[13] Trelford, J. D., Anderson, D. G., Hanson, F. W., Mendel, V. & Sawyer, R. H. (1972) Amnion autografts and allografts as a cover for skin defects in sheep. A preliminary report. *J Med, 3*, 81-7.

[14] Trelford, J. D., Hanson, F. W., Anderson, D. G. & Mendel, V. E. (1975) Amnion autografts, permanent structure. *J Med, 6*, 243-7.

[15] Robson, M. C., Samburg, J. L. & Krizek, T. J. (1972) Quantitative comparison of biological dressings. *Surg Forum, 23*, 503-5.

[16] Robson, M. C., Krizek, T. J., Koss, N. & Samburg, J. L. (1973) Amniotic membranes as a temporary wound dressing. *Surg Gynecol Obstet, 136*, 904-6.

[17] Robson, M. C. & Krizek, T. J. (1974) Clinical experiences with amniotic membranes as a temporary biologic dressing. *Conn Med, 38*, 449-51.

[18] Colocho, G., Graham, W. P., 3rd, Greene, A. E., Matheson, D. W. & Lynch, D. (1974) Human amniotic membrane as a physiologic wound dressing. *Arch Surg, 109*, 370-3.

[19] Gruss, J. S. & Jirsch, D. W. (1978) Human amniotic membrane: a versatile wound dressing. *Can Med Assoc J, 118*, 1237-46.

[20] Kesting, M. R., Wolff, K. D., Hohlweg-Majert, B. & Steinstraesser, L. (2008) The role of allogenic amniotic membrane in burn treatment. *J Burn Care Res, 29*, 907-16.

[21] Haberal, M., Oner, Z., Bayraktar, U. & Bilgin, N. (1987) The use of silver nitrate-incorporated amniotic membrane as a temporary dressing. *Burns Incl Therm Inj, 13*, 159-63.

[22] Haberal, M., Oner, Z. & Bayraktar, U. (1987) Analysis of 745 hospitalized burn patients. *Ann Med Burn Club, 10*, 45-48.

[23] Lorusso, R., Geraci, V. & Masellis, M. (1989) The treatment of superficial burns with biological and synthetic material: frozen amnion and biobrane. *Ann Med Burn Club, 2*, 79-84.

[24] Sawhney, C. P. (1989) Amniotic membrane as a biological dressing in the management of burns. *Burns, 15*, 339-42.

[25] Subrahmanyam, M. (1994) Honey-impregnated gauze versus amniotic membrane in the treatment of burns. *Burns, 20*, 331-3.

[26] Ugar, N. & Haberal, M. (1994) Comparison of various dressing materials used for out-patient burn treatment at our centre. *Ann Med Burn Club, 7*, 147-149.

[27] Ravishanker, R., Bath, A. S. & Roy, R. (2003) "Amnion Bank"--the use of long term glycerol preserved amniotic membranes in the management of superficial and superficial partial thickness burns. *Burns, 29*, 369-74.

[28] Singh, R., Kumar, D., Kumar, P. & Chacharkar, M. P. (2008) Development and evaluation of silver-impregnated amniotic membrane as an antimicrobial burn dressing. *J Burn Care Res, 29*, 64-72.

[29] Ramakrishnan, K. M. & Jayaraman, V. (1997) Management of partial-thickness burn wounds by amniotic membrane: a cost-effective treatment in developing countries. *Burns, 23 Suppl 1*, S33-6.

[30] Gajiwala, K. & Gajiwala, A. L. (2004) Evaluation of lyophilised, gamma-irradiated amnion as a biological dressing. *Cell Tissue Bank, 5*, 73-80.

[31] Singh, R., Purohit, S., Chacharkar, M. P., Bhandari, P. S. & Bath, A. S. (2007) Microbiological safety and clinical efficacy of radiation sterilized amniotic membranes for treatment of second-degree burns. *Burns, 33*, 505-10.

[32] Gajiwala, K. & Lobo Gajiwala, A. (2003) Use of banked tissue in plastic surgery. *Cell Tissue Bank, 4*, 141-6.

[33] Maral, T., Borman, H., Arslan, H., Demirhan, B., Akinbingol, G. & Haberal, M. (1999) Effectiveness of human amnion preserved long-term in glycerol as a temporary biological dressing. *Burns, 25*, 625-35.

[34] Atanassov, W., Mazgalova, J. & Todorov, R. (1994) Use of human amniotic membranes as biological dressings in contemporary treatment of burns. *Ann Med Burn Club, 7*, 202-205.

[35] Hadjiiski, O. & Atanassov, N. (1996) Amniotic membranes for temporary burn coverage. *Ann Burns Fire Disasters, 9*, 88-92.

[36] Bari, M., Choudhury, M. & Khan, A. (2002) Role of human foetal membranes (amniotic membrane) in the management of burn wounds. *Ann Burns Fire Disasters, 15*, 183-186.

[37] Dino, B. R., Eufemio, G. G. & De Villa, M. S. (1966) Human amnion : the establishment of an amnion bank and its practical applications in surgery. *J Philipp Med Assoc, 42*, 357-66.

[38] Quinby, W. C., Jr., Hoover, H. C., Scheflan, M., Walters, P. T., Slavin, S. A. & Bondoc, C. C. (1982) Clinical trials of amniotic membranes in burn wound care. *Plast Reconstr Surg, 70*, 711-17.

[39] Rao, T. V. & Chandrasekharam, V. (1981) Use of dry human and bovine amnion as a biological dressing. *Arch Surg, 116*, 891-6.

[40] Subrahmanyam, M. (1995) Amniotic membrane as a cover for microskin grafts. *Br J Plast Surg, 48*, 477-8.

[41] Branski, L. K., Herndon, D. N., Celis, M. M., Norbury, W. B., Masters, O. E. & Jeschke, M. G. (2008) Amnion in the treatment of pediatric partial-thickness facial burns. *Burns, 34*, 393-9.

[42] Faulk, W. P., Matthews, R., Stevens, P. J., Bennett, J. P., Burgos, H. & Hsi, B. L. (1980) Human amnion as an adjunct in wound healing. *Lancet, 1*, 1156-8.

[43] Bennett, J. P., Matthews, R. & Faulk, W. P. (1980) Treatment of chronic ulceration of the legs with human amnion. *Lancet, 1*, 1153-6.

[44] Ward, D. J. & Bennett, J. P. (1984) The long-term results of the use of human amnion in the treatment of leg ulcers. *Br J Plast Surg, 37*, 191-3.

[45] Ward, D. J., Bennett, J. P., Burgos, H. & Fabre, J. (1989) The healing of chronic venous leg ulcers with prepared human amnion. *Br J Plast Surg, 42*, 463-7.

[46] Singh, R., Chouhan, U. S., Purohit, S., Gupta, P., Kumar, P., Kumar, A., Chacharkar, M. P., Kachhawa, D. & Ghiya, B. C. (2004) Radiation processed amniotic membranes in the treatment of non-healing ulcers of different etiologies. *Cell Tissue Bank, 5*, 129-34.

[47] Mermet, I., Pottier, N., Sainthillier, J. M., Malugani, C., Cairey-Remonnay, S., Maddens, S., Riethmuller, D., Tiberghien, P., Humbert, P. & Aubin, F. (2007) Use of amniotic membrane transplantation in the treatment of venous leg ulcers. *Wound Repair Regen, 15*, 459-64.

[48] Brindeau, A. (1934) Création d'un vagin artificiel à l'aide des membranes ovulaires d'un oeuf à terme. *Gynecol Obstet (Paris), 29*, 385.

[49] Burger, K. (1947) Weitere Erfahrungen uber die kunsliche Scheidenbildung mit Eihauten. *Zentralbl Gynaekol, 69*, 1153.

[50] Trelford, J. D., Hanson, F. W. & Anderson, D. G. (1973) Amniotic membrane as a living surgical dressing in human patients. *Oncology, 28*, 358-64.

[51] Dhall, K. (1984) Amnion graft for treatment of congenital absence of the vagina. *Br J Obstet Gynaecol, 91*, 279-82.

[52] Nisolle, M. & Donnez, J. (1992) Vaginoplasty using amniotic membranes in cases of vaginal agenesis or after vaginectomy. *J Gynecol Surg, 8*, 25-30.

[53] Ghanbari, Z., Dahaghin, M. & Borna, S. (2006) Long-term outcomes of vaginal reconstruction with and without amnion grafts. *Int J Gynaecol Obstet, 92*, 163-4.

[54] Fotopoulou, C., Sehouli, J., Gehrmann, N., Schoenborn, I. & Lichtenegger, W. (2009) Functional and anatomic results of amnion vaginoplasty in young women with Mayer-Rokitansky-Kuster-Hauser syndrome. *Fertil Steril*.

[55] Brandt, F. T., Albuquerque, C. D. & Lorenzato, F. R. (2000) Female urethral reconstruction with amnion grafts. *Int J Surg Investig, 1*, 409-14.

[56] Massee, J., RE, S., Dockerty, M. & Gallenback, G. (1962) Use of fetal membranes as replacement for pelvic peritoneum after pelvic exenteration in the dog. *Gynecol Obstet, 13*, 407.

[57] Trelford-Sauder, M., Trelford, J. D. & Matolo, N. M. (1977) Replacement of the peritoneum with amnion following pelvic exenteration. *Surg Gynecol Obstet, 145*, 699-701.

[58] Trelford-Sauder, M., Dawe, E. J. & Trelford, J. D. (1978) Use of allograft amniotic membrane for control of intra-abdominal adhesions. *J Med, 9*, 273-84.

[59] Young, R. L., Cota, J., Zund, G., Mason, B. A. & Wheeler, J. M. (1991) The use of an amniotic membrane graft to prevent postoperative adhesions. *Fertil Steril, 55*, 624-8.

[60] Kelekci, S., Uygur, D., Yilmaz, B., Sut, N. & Yesildaglar, N. (2007) Comparison of human amniotic membrane and hyaluronate/carboxymethylcellulose membrane for prevention of adhesion formation in rats. *Arch Gynecol Obstet, 276*, 355-9.

[61] Rennekampff, H. O., Dohrmann, P., Fory, R. & Fandrich, F. (1994) Evaluation of amniotic membrane as adhesion prophylaxis in a novel surgical gastroschisis model. *J Invest Surg, 7*, 187-93.

[62] Szabo, A., Haj, M., Waxsman, I. & Eitan, A. (2000) Evaluation of seprafilm and amniotic membrane as adhesion prophylaxis in mesh repair of abdominal wall hernia in rats. *Eur Surg Res, 32*, 125-8.

[63] Badawy, S. Z., Baggish, M. S., ElBakry, M. M. & Baltoyannis, P. (1989) Evaluation of tissue healing and adhesion formation after an intraabdominal amniotic membrane graft in the rat. *J Reprod Med, 34*, 198-202.

[64] Arora, M., Jaroudi, K. A., Hamilton, C. J. & Dayel, F. (1994) Controlled comparison of interceed and amniotic membrane graft in the prevention of postoperative adhesions in the rabbit uterine horn model. *Eur J Obstet Gynecol Reprod Biol, 55*, 179-82.

[65] Muralidharan, S., Gu, J., Laub, G. W., Cichon, R., Daloisio, C. & McGrath, L. B. (1991) A new biological membrane for pericardial closure. *J Biomed Mater Res, 25*, 1201-9.

[66] Ozgenel, G. Y. (2004) The effects of a combination of hyaluronic and amniotic membrane on the formation of peritendinous adhesions after flexor tendon surgery in chickens. *J Bone Joint Surg Br, 86*, 301-7.

[67] Ozgenel, G. Y. & Filiz, G. (2004) Combined application of human amniotic membrane wrapping and hyaluronic acid injection in epineurectomized rat sciatic nerve. *J Reconstr Microsurg, 20*, 153-7.

[68] Demirkan, F., Colakoglu, N., Herek, O. & Erkula, G. (2002) The use of amniotic membrane in flexor tendon repair: an experimental model. *Arch Orthop Trauma Surg, 122*, 396-9.

[69] Lawson, V. G. (1985) Oral cavity reconstruction using pectoralis major muscle and amnion. *Arch Otolaryngol, 111*, 230-3.

[70] Zohar, Y., Talmi, Y. P., Finkelstein, Y., Shvili, Y., Sadov, R. & Laurian, N. (1987) Use of human amniotic membrane in otolaryngologic practice. *Laryngoscope, 97*, 978-80.

[71] Guler, R., Ercan, M. T., Ulutuncel, N., Devrim, H. & Uran, N. (1997) Measurement of blood flow by the 133Xe clearance technique to grafts of amnion used in vestibuloplasty. *Br J Oral Maxillofac Surg, 35*, 280-3.

[72] Samandari, M. H., Yaghmaei, M., Ejlali, M., Moshref, M. & Saffar, A. S. (2004) Use of amnion as a graft material in vestibuloplasty: a preliminary report. *Oral Surg Oral Med Oral Pathol Oral Radiol Endod, 97*, 574-8.

[73] Kim, J. C. & Tseng, S. C. (1995) Transplantation of preserved human amniotic membrane for surface reconstruction in severely damaged rabbit corneas. *Cornea, 14*, 473-84.

[74] Meller, D. & Tseng, S. C. (1999) Conjunctival epithelial cell differentiation on amniotic membrane. *Invest Ophthalmol Vis Sci, 40*, 878-86.

[75] Sippel, K. C., Ma, J. J. & Foster, C. S. (2001) Amniotic membrane surgery. *Curr Opin Ophthalmol, 12*, 269-81.

[76] Szurman, P., Warga, M., Grisanti, S., Roters, S., Rohrbach, J. M., Aisenbrey, S., Kaczmarek, R. T. & Bartz-Schmidt, K. U. (2006) Sutureless amniotic membrane fixation using fibrin glue for ocular surface reconstruction in a rabbit model. *Cornea, 25*, 460-6.

[77] Solomon, A., Meller, D. & Prabhasawat, P. (2001) Amniotic membrane grafts for non-traumatic corneal perforations, descemetoceles and deep ulcers. *Ophthalmology, 109*, 694-703.

[78] Azuara-Blanco, A., Pillai, C. T. & Dua, H. S. (1999) Amniotic membrane transplantation for ocular surface reconstruction. *Br J Ophthalmol, 83*, 399-402.

[79] Letko, E., Stechschulte, S. U., Kenyon, K. R., Sadeq, N., Romero, T. R., Samson, C. M., Nguyen, Q. D., Harper, S. L., Primack, J. D., Azar, D. T., Gruterich, M., Dohlman, C. H., Baltatzis, S. & Foster, C. S. (2001) Amniotic membrane inlay and overlay grafting for corneal epithelial defects and stromal ulcers. *Arch Ophthalmol, 119*, 659-63.

[80] Uhlig, C. E., Busse, H. & Groppe, M. (2006) Use of fibrin glue in fixation of amniotic membranes in sterile corneal ulceration. *Am J Ophthalmol, 142*, 189-91.

[81] Meller, D., Pires, R. T., Mack, R. J., Figueiredo, F., Heiligenhaus, A., Park, W. C., Prabhasawat, P., John, T., McLeod, S. D., Steuhl, K. P. & Tseng, S. C. (2000) Amniotic membrane transplantation for acute chemical or thermal burns. *Ophthalmology, 107*, 980-9; discussion 990.

[82] Park, W. C. & Tseng, S. C. (2000) Modulation of acute inflammation and keratocyte death by suturing, blood, and amniotic membrane in PRK. *Invest Ophthalmol Vis Sci, 41*, 2906-14.

[83] Kheirkhah, A., Johnson, D. A., Paranjpe, D. R., Raju, V. K., Casas, V. & Tseng, S. C. (2008) Temporary sutureless amniotic membrane patch for acute alkaline burns. *Arch Ophthalmol, 126*, 1059-66.

[84] Joseph, A., Dua, H. S. & King, A. J. (2001) Failure of amniotic membrane transplantation in the treatment of acute ocular burns. *Br J Ophthalmol, 85*, 1065-9.

[85] John, T., Foulks, G. N., John, M. E., Cheng, K. & Hu, D. (2002) Amniotic membrane in the surgical management of acute toxic epidermal necrolysis. *Ophthalmology, 109*, 351-60.

[86] Shimazaki, J., Kosaka, K., Shimmura, S. & Tsubota, K. (2003) Amniotic membrane transplantation with conjunctival autograft for recurrent pterygium. *Ophthalmology, 110*, 119-24.

[87] Ma, D. H., See, L. C., Liau, S. B. & Tsai, R. J. (2000) Amniotic membrane graft for primary pterygium: comparison with conjunctival autograft and topical mitomycin C treatment. *Br J Ophthalmol, 84*, 973-8.

[88] Prabhasawat, P., Barton, K., Burkett, G. & Tseng, S. C. (1997) Comparison of conjunctival autografts, amniotic membrane grafts, and primary closure for pterygium excision. *Ophthalmology, 104*, 974-85.

[89] Solomon, A., Pires, R. T. & Tseng, S. C. (2001) Amniotic membrane transplantation after extensive removal of primary and recurrent pterygia. *Ophthalmology, 108*, 449-60.

[90] Luanratanakorn, P., Ratanapakorn, T., Suwan-Apichon, O. & Chuck, R. S. (2006) Randomised controlled study of conjunctival autograft versus amniotic membrane graft in pterygium excision. *Br J Ophthalmol, 90*, 1476-80.

[91] Tananuvat, N. & Martin, T. (2004) The results of amniotic membrane transplantation for primary pterygium compared with conjunctival autograft. *Cornea, 23*, 458-63.

[92] Paridaens, D., Beekhuis, H., van Den Bosch, W., Remeyer, L. & Melles, G. (2001) Amniotic membrane transplantation in the management of conjunctival malignant melanoma and primary acquired melanosis with atypia. *Br J Ophthalmol, 85*, 658-61.

[93] Solomon, A., Espana, E. M. & Tseng, S. C. (2003) Amniotic membrane transplantation for reconstruction of the conjunctival fornices. *Ophthalmology, 110*, 93-100.

[94] Tseng, S. C., Di Pascuale, M. A., Liu, D. T., Gao, Y. Y. & Baradaran-Rafii, A. (2005) Intraoperative mitomycin C and amniotic membrane transplantation for fornix reconstruction in severe cicatricial ocular surface diseases. *Ophthalmology, 112*, 896-903.

[95] Budenz, D. L., Barton, K. & Tseng, S. C. (2000) Amniotic membrane transplantation for repair of leaking glaucoma filtering blebs. *Am J Ophthalmol, 130*, 580-8.

[96] Hanada, K., Shimazaki, J., Shimmura, S. & Tsubota, K. (2001) Multilayered amniotic membrane transplantation for severe ulceration of the cornea and sclera. *Am J Ophthalmol, 131*, 324-31.

[97] Kruse, F. E., Rohrschneider, K. & Volcker, H. E. (1999) Multilayer amniotic membrane transplantation for reconstruction of deep corneal ulcers. *Ophthalmology, 106*, 1504-10; discussion 1511.

[98] Rodriguez-Ares, M. T., Tourino, R., Lopez-Valladares, M. J. & Gude, F. (2004) Multilayer amniotic membrane transplantation in the treatment of corneal perforations. *Cornea, 23*, 577-83.

[99] Hick, S., Demers, P. E., Brunette, I., La, C., Mabon, M. & Duchesne, B. (2005) Amniotic membrane transplantation and fibrin glue in the management of corneal ulcers and perforations: a review of 33 cases. *Cornea, 24*, 369-77.

[100] Lee, S. H. & Tseng, S. C. (1997) Amniotic membrane transplantation for persistent epithelial defects with ulceration. *Am J Ophthalmol, 123*, 303-12.

[101] Espana, E. M., Grueterich, M., Sandoval, H., Solomon, A., Alfonso, E., Karp, C. L., Fantes, F. & Tseng, S. C. (2003) Amniotic membrane transplantation for bullous keratopathy in eyes with poor visual potential. *J Cataract Refract Surg, 29*, 279-84.

[102] Pires, R. T., Tseng, S. C., Prabhasawat, P., Puangsricharern, V., Maskin, S. L., Kim, J. C. & Tan, D. T. (1999) Amniotic membrane transplantation for symptomatic bullous keratopathy. *Arch Ophthalmol, 117*, 1291-7.

[103] Anderson, D. F., Prabhasawat, P., Alfonso, E. & Tseng, S. C. (2001) Amniotic membrane transplantation after the primary surgical management of band keratopathy. *Cornea, 20*, 354-61.

[104] Schwab, I. R., Reyes, M. & Isseroff, R. R. (2000) Successful transplantation of bioengineered tissue replacements in patients with ocular surface disease. *Cornea, 19*, 421-6.

[105] Tsai, R. J., Li, L. M. & Chen, J. K. (2000) Reconstruction of damaged corneas by transplantation of autologous limbal epithelial cells. *N Engl J Med, 343*, 86-93.

[106] Nakamura, T., Endo, K., Cooper, L. J., Fullwood, N. J., Tanifuji, N., Tsuzuki, M., Koizumi, N., Inatomi, T., Sano, Y. & Kinoshita, S. (2003) The successful culture and autologous transplantation of rabbit oral mucosal epithelial cells on amniotic membrane. *Invest Ophthalmol Vis Sci, 44*, 106-16.

[107] Inatomi, T., Nakamura, T., Koizumi, N., Sotozono, C., Yokoi, N. & Kinoshita, S. (2006) Midterm results on ocular surface reconstruction using cultivated autologous oral mucosal epithelial transplantation. *Am J Ophthalmol, 141*, 267-275.

[108] Inatomi, T., Nakamura, T., Kojyo, M., Koizumi, N., Sotozono, C. & Kinoshita, S. (2006) Ocular surface reconstruction with combination of cultivated autologous oral mucosal epithelial transplantation and penetrating keratoplasty. *Am J Ophthalmol, 142*, 757-64.

[109] Adds, P. J., Hunt, C. & Hartley, S. (2001) Bacterial contamination of amniotic membrane. *Br J Ophthalmol, 85*, 228-30.

[110] Tsubota, K., Satake, Y., Ohyama, M., Toda, I., Takano, Y., Ono, M., Shinozaki, N. & Shimazaki, J. (1996) Surgical reconstruction of the ocular surface in advanced ocular cicatricial pemphigoid and Stevens-Johnson syndrome. *Am J Ophthalmol, 122*, 38-52.

[111] Hennerbichler, S., Reichl, B., Pleiner, D., Gabriel, C., Eibl, J. & Redl, H. (2006) The influence of various storage conditions on cell viability in amniotic membrane. *Cell Tissue Bank.*

[112] Parolini, O., Alviano, F., Bagnara, G. P., Bilic, G., Buhring, H. J., Evangelista, M., Hennerbichler, S., Liu, B., Magatti, M., Mao, N., Miki, T., Marongiu, F., Nakajima, H., Nikaido, T., Portmann-Lanz, C. B.,

Sankar, V., Soncini, M., Stadler, G., Surbek, D., Takahashi, T. A., Redl, H., Sakuragawa, N., Wolbank, S., Zeisberger, S., Zisch, A. & Strom, S. C. (2008) Concise review: isolation and characterization of cells from human term placenta: outcome of the first international Workshop on Placenta Derived Stem Cells. *Stem Cells, 26*, 300-11.

[113] Parolini, O., Soncini, M., Evangelista, M. & Schmidt, D. (2009) Amniotic membrane and amniotic fluid-derived cells: potential tools for regenerative medicine? *Regen Med, 4*, 275-91.

[114] Sankar, V. & Muthusamy, R. (2003) Role of human amniotic epithelial cell transplantation in spinal cord injury repair research. *Neuroscience, 118*, 11-7.

[115] Zhao, P., Ise, H., Hongo, M., Ota, M., Konishi, I. & Nikaido, T. (2005) Human amniotic mesenchymal cells have some characteristics of cardiomyocytes. *Transplantation, 79*, 528-35.

[116] Meng, X. T., Li, C., Dong, Z. Y., Liu, J. M., Li, W., Liu, Y., Xue, H. & Chen, D. (2008) Co-transplantation of bFGF-expressing amniotic epithelial cells and neural stem cells promotes functional recovery in spinal cord-injured rats. *Cell Biol Int, 32*, 1546-58.

[117] Kong, X. Y., Cai, Z., Pan, L., Zhang, L., Shu, J., Dong, Y. L., Yang, N., Li, Q., Huang, X. J. & Zuo, P. P. (2008) Transplantation of human amniotic cells exerts neuroprotection in MPTP-induced Parkinson disease mice. *Brain Res, 1205*, 108-15.

[118] Liu, T., Wu, J., Huang, Q., Hou, Y., Jiang, Z., Zang, S. & Guo, L. (2008) Human amniotic epithelial cells ameliorate behavioral dysfunction and reduce infarct size in the rat middle cerebral artery occlusion model. *Shock, 29*, 603-11.

[119] Bailo, M., Soncini, M., Vertua, E., Signoroni, P. B., Sanzone, S., Lombardi, G., Arienti, D., Calamani, F., Zatti, D., Paul, P., Albertini, A., Zorzi, F., Cavagnini, A., Candotti, F., Wengler, G. S. & Parolini, O. (2004) Engraftment potential of human amnion and chorion cells derived from term placenta. *Transplantation, 78*, 1439-48.

[120] Marcus, A. J., Coyne, T. M., Rauch, J., Woodbury, D. & Black, I. B. (2008) Isolation, characterization, and differentiation of stem cells derived from the rat amniotic membrane. *Differentiation, 76*, 130-44.

[121] Chen, C. P., Liu, S. H., Huang, J. P., Aplin, J. D., Wu, Y. H., Chen, P. C., Hu, C. S., Ko, C. C., Lee, M. Y. & Chen, C. Y. (2009) Engraftment potential of human placenta-derived mesenchymal stem cells after in utero transplantation in rats. *Hum Reprod, 24*, 154-65.

[122] Brooke, G., Tong, H., Levesque, J. P. & Atkinson, K. (2008) Molecular trafficking mechanisms of multipotent mesenchymal stem cells derived from human bone marrow and placenta. *Stem Cells Dev, 17*, 929-40.

[123] Sakuragawa, N., Thangavel, R., Mizuguchi, M., Hirasawa, M. & Kamo, I. (1996) Expression of markers for both neuronal and glial cells in human amniotic epithelial cells. *Neurosci Lett, 209*, 9-12.

[124] Elwan, M. A., Thangavel, R., Ono, F. & Sakuragawa, N. (1998) Synthesis and release of catecholamines by cultured monkey amniotic epithelial cells. *J Neurosci Res, 53*, 107-13.

[125] Okawa, H., Okuda, O., Arai, H., Sakuragawa, N. & Sato, K. (2001) Amniotic epithelial cells transform into neuron-like cells in the ischemic brain. *Neuroreport, 12*, 4003-7.

[126] Sakuragawa, N., Misawa, H., Ohsugi, K., Kakishita, K., Ishii, T., Thangavel, R., Tohyama, J., Elwan, M., Yokoyama, Y., Okuda, O., Arai, H., Ogino, I. & Sato, K. (1997) Evidence for active acetylcholine metabolism in human amniotic epithelial cells: applicable to intracerebral allografting for neurologic disease. *Neurosci Lett, 232*, 53-6.

[127] Elwan, M. A. & Sakuragawa, N. (1997) Evidence for synthesis and release of catecholamines by human amniotic epithelial cells. *Neuroreport, 8*, 3435-8.

[128] Ishii, T., Ohsugi, K., Nakamura, S., Sato, K., Hashimoto, M., Mikoshiba, K. & Sakuragawa, N. (1999) Gene expression of oligodendrocyte markers in human amniotic epithelial cells using neural cell-type-specific expression system. *Neurosci Lett, 268*, 131-4.

[129] Uchida, S., Inanaga, Y., Kobayashi, M., Hurukawa, S., Araie, M. & Sakuragawa, N. (2000) Neurotrophic function of conditioned medium from human amniotic epithelial cells. *J Neurosci Res, 62*, 585-90.

[130] Koyano, S., Fukui, A., Uchida, S., Yamada, K., Asashima, M. & Sakuragawa, N. (2002) Synthesis and release of activin and noggin by cultured human amniotic epithelial cells. *Dev Growth Differ, 44*, 103-12.

[131] Sakuragawa, N., Kakinuma, K., Kikuchi, A., Okano, H., Uchida, S., Kamo, I., Kobayashi, M. & Yokoyama, Y. (2004) Human amnion mesenchyme cells express phenotypes of neuroglial progenitor cells. *J Neurosci Res, 78*, 208-14.

[132] Tcheng, M., Oliver, L., Courtois, Y. & Jeanny, J. C. (1994) Effects of exogenous FGFs on growth, differentiation, and survival of chick neural retina cells. *Exp Cell Res, 212*, 30-5.

[133] Meng, X. T., Chen, D., Dong, Z. Y. & Liu, J. M. (2007) Enhanced neural differentiation of neural stem cells and neurite growth by amniotic epithelial cell co-culture. *Cell Biol Int, 31*, 691-8.

[134] Schroeder, A., Theiss, C., Steuhl, K. P., Meller, K. & Meller, D. (2007) Effects of the human amniotic membrane on axonal outgrowth of dorsal root ganglia neurons in culture. *Curr Eye Res, 32*, 731-8.

[135] Portmann-Lanz, C. B., Schoeberlein, A., Huber, A., Sager, R., Malek, A., Holzgreve, W. & Surbek, D. V. (2006) Placental mesenchymal stem cells as potential autologous graft for pre- and perinatal neuroregeneration. *Am J Obstet Gynecol, 194*, 664-73.

[136] Yu, S. J., Soncini, M., Kaneko, Y., Hess, D. C., Parolini, O. & Borlongan, C. V. (2009) Amnion: a potent graft source for cell therapy in stroke. *Cell Transplant, 18*, 111-8.

[137] Kakishita, K., Elwan, M. A., Nakao, N., Itakura, T. & Sakuragawa, N. (2000) Human amniotic epithelial cells produce dopamine and survive after implantation into the striatum of a rat model of Parkinson's disease: a potential source of donor for transplantation therapy. *Exp Neurol, 165*, 27-34.

[138] Kakishita, K., Nakao, N., Sakuragawa, N. & Itakura, T. (2003) Implantation of human amniotic epithelial cells prevents the degeneration of nigral dopamine neurons in rats with 6-hydroxydopamine lesions. *Brain Res, 980*, 48-56.

[139] Kosuga, M., Takahashi, S., Tanabe, A., Fujino, M., Li, X. K., Suzuki, S., Yamada, M., Kakishita, K., Ono, F., Sakuragawa, N. & Okuyama, T. (2001) Widespread distribution of adenovirus-transduced monkey amniotic epithelial cells after local intracerebral injection: implication for cell-mediated therapy for lysosome storage disorders. *Cell Transplant, 10*, 435-9.

[140] Ilancheran, S., Michalska, A., Peh, G., Wallace, E. M., Pera, M. & Manuelpillai, U. (2007) Stem Cells Derived from Human Fetal Membranes Display Multi-Lineage Differentiation Potential. *Biol Reprod, 77*, 577-588.

[141] Ventura, C., Cantoni, S., Bianchi, F., Lionetti, V., Cavallini, C., Scarlata, I., Foroni, L., Maioli, M., Bonsi, L., Alviano, F., Fossati, V., Bagnara, G. P., Pasquinelli, G., Recchia, F. A. & Perbellini, A. (2007)

Hyaluronan Mixed Esters of Butyric and Retinoic Acid Drive Cardiac and Endothelial Fate in Term Placenta Human Mesenchymal Stem Cells and Enhance Cardiac Repair in Infarcted Rat Hearts. *J Biol Chem, 282*, 14243-14252.

[142] Okamoto, K., Miyoshi, S., Toyoda, M., Hida, N., Ikegami, Y., Makino, H., Nishiyama, N., Tsuji, H., Cui, C. H., Segawa, K., Uyama, T., Kami, D., Miyado, K., Asada, H., Matsumoto, K., Saito, H., Yoshimura, Y., Ogawa, S., Aeba, R., Yozu, R. & Umezawa, A. (2007) 'Working' cardiomyocytes exhibiting plateau action potentials from human placenta-derived extraembryonic mesodermal cells. *Exp Cell Res, 313*, 2550-62.

[143] Alviano, F., Fossati, V., Marchionni, C., Arpinati, M., Bonsi, L., Franchina, M., Lanzoni, G., Cantoni, S., Cavallini, C., Bianchi, F., Tazzari, P. L., Pasquinelli, G., Foroni, L., Ventura, C., Grossi, A. & Bagnara, G. P. (2007) Term Amniotic membrane is a high throughput source for multipotent Mesenchymal Stem Cells with the ability to differentiate into endothelial cells in vitro. *BMC Dev Biol, 7*, 11.

[144] Wu, C. C., Chao, Y. C., Chen, C. N., Chien, S., Chen, Y. C., Chien, C. C., Chiu, J. J. & Linju Yen, B. (2008) Synergism of biochemical and mechanical stimuli in the differentiation of human placenta-derived multipotent cells into endothelial cells. *J Biomech, 41*, 813-21.

[145] Sakuragawa, N., Enosawa, S., Ishii, T., Thangavel, R., Tashiro, T., Okuyama, T. & Suzuki, S. (2000) Human amniotic epithelial cells are promising transgene carriers for allogeneic cell transplantation into liver. *J Hum Genet, 45*, 171-6.

[146] Takashima, S., Ise, H., Zhao, P., Akaike, T. & Nikaido, T. (2004) Human amniotic epithelial cells possess hepatocyte-like characteristics and functions. *Cell Struct Funct, 29*, 73-84.

[147] Miki, T., Lehmann, T., Cai, H., Stolz, D. B. & Strom, S. C. (2005) Stem cell characteristics of amniotic epithelial cells. *Stem Cells, 23*, 1549-59.

[148] Scaggiante, B., Pineschi, A., Sustersich, M., Andolina, M., Agosti, E. & Romeo, D. (1987) Successful therapy of Niemann-Pick disease by implantation of human amniotic membrane. *Transplantation, 44*, 59-61.

[149] Scaggiante, B., Comelli, M. & Romeo, D. (1991) Secretion of lysosomal hydrolases by cultured human amnion epithelial cells. *Exp Cell Res, 195*, 194-8.

[150] Bembi, B., Comelli, M., Scaggiante, B., Pineschi, A., Rapelli, S., Gornati, R., Montorfano, G., Berra, B., Agosti, E. & Romeo, D. (1992)

Treatment of sphingomyelinase deficiency by repeated implantations of amniotic epithelial cells. *Am J Med Genet, 44*, 527-33.

[151] Wei, J. P., Zhang, T. S., Kawa, S., Aizawa, T., Ota, M., Akaike, T., Kato, K., Konishi, I. & Nikaido, T. (2003) Human amnion-isolated cells normalize blood glucose in streptozotocin-induced diabetic mice. *Cell Transplant, 12*, 545-52.

[152] Chang, C. M., Kao, C. L., Chang, Y. L., Yang, M. J., Chen, Y. C., Sung, B. L., Tsai, T. H., Chao, K. C., Chiou, S. H. & Ku, H. H. (2007) Placenta-derived multipotent stem cells induced to differentiate into insulin-positive cells. *Biochem Biophys Res Commun, 357*, 414-20.

[153] Cargnoni, A., Gibelli, L., Tosini, A., Signoroni, P. B., Nassuato, C., Arienti, D., Lombardi, G., Albertini, A., Wengler, G. S. & Parolini, O. (2009) Transplantation of allogeneic and xenogeneic placenta-derived cells reduces bleomycin-induced lung fibrosis. *Cell Transplant*, *18*, 405-22.

[154] Medawar, P. (1953) Some immunological and endocrinological problems raised by the evolution of viviparity in vertebrates. *Symp Soc Exp Biol, 7*, 320-338.

[155] von Rango, U. (2008) Fetal tolerance in human pregnancy--a crucial balance between acceptance and limitation of trophoblast invasion. *Immunol Lett, 115*, 21-32.

[156] Koch, C. A. & Platt, J. L. (2007) T cell recognition and immunity in the fetus and mother. *Cell Immunol, 248*, 12-7.

[157] Aluvihare, V. R., Kallikourdis, M. & Betz, A. G. (2005) Tolerance, suppression and the fetal allograft. *J Mol Med, 83*, 88-96.

[158] Trelford, J. D. & Trelford-Sauder, M. (1979) The amnion in surgery, past and present. *Am J Obstet Gynecol, 134*, 833-45.

[159] Adinolfi, M., Akle, C. A., McColl, I., Fensom, A. H., Tansley, L., Connolly, P., Hsi, B. L., Faulk, W. P., Travers, P. & Bodmer, W. F. (1982) Expression of HLA antigens, beta 2-microglobulin and enzymes by human amniotic epithelial cells. *Nature, 295*, 325-7.

[160] Kubo, M., Sonoda, Y., Muramatsu, R. & Usui, M. (2001) Immunogenicity of human amniotic membrane in experimental xenotransplantation. *Invest Ophthalmol Vis Sci, 42*, 1539-46.

[161] Li, H., Niederkorn, J. Y., Neelam, S., Mayhew, E., Word, R. A., McCulley, J. P. & Alizadeh, H. (2005) Immunosuppressive factors secreted by human amniotic epithelial cells. *Invest Ophthalmol Vis Sci, 46*, 900-7.

[162] Magatti, M., De Munari, S., Vertua, E., Gibelli, L., Wengler, G. S. & Parolini, O. (2008) Human amnion mesenchyme harbors cells with allogeneic T-cell suppression and stimulation capabilities. *Stem Cells, 26*, 182-92.

[163] Wolbank, S., Peterbauer, A., Fahrner, M., Hennerbichler, S., van Griensven, M., Stadler, G., Redl, H. & Gabriel, C. (2007) Dose-Dependent Immunomodulatory Effect of Human Stem Cells from Amniotic Membrane: A Comparison with Human Mesenchymal Stem Cells from Adipose Tissue. *Tissue Eng, 13*, 1173-83.

[164] Wolbank, S., Stadler, G., Peterbauer, A., Gillich, A., Karbiener, M., Streubel, B., Wieser, M., Katinger, H., van Griensven, M., Redl, H., Gabriel, C., Grillari, J. & Grillari-Voglauer, R. (2009) Telomerase Immortalized Human Amnion- and Adipose-Derived Mesenchymal Stem Cells: Maintenance of Differentiation and Immunomodulatory Characteristics. *Tissue Eng Part A*.

[165] Magatti, M., De Munari, S., Vertua, E., Nassuato, C., Albertini, A., Wengler, G. S. & Parolini, O. (2009) Amniotic mesenchymal tissue cells inhibit dendritic cell differentiation of peripheral blood and amnion resident monocytes. *Cell Transplant*.

[166] Shimazaki, J., Yang, H. Y. & Tsubota, K. (1997) Amniotic membrane transplantation for ocular surface reconstruction in patients with chemical and thermal burns. *Ophthalmology, 104*, 2068-76.

[167] Choi, Y. S., Kim, J. Y., Wee, W. R. & Lee, J. H. (1998) Effect of the application of human amniotic membrane on rabbit corneal wound healing after excimer laser photorefractive keratectomy. *Cornea, 17*, 389-95.

[168] Lee, S. B., Li, D. Q., Tan, D. T., Meller, D. C. & Tseng, S. C. (2000) Suppression of TGF-beta signaling in both normal conjunctival fibroblasts and pterygial body fibroblasts by amniotic membrane. *Curr Eye Res, 20*, 325-34.

[169] Shimmura, S., Shimazaki, J., Ohashi, Y. & Tsubota, K. (2001) Antiinflammatory effects of amniotic membrane transplantation in ocular surface disorders. *Cornea, 20*, 408-13.

[170] Solomon, A., Wajngarten, M., Alviano, F., Anteby, I., Elchalal, U., Pe'er, J. & Levi-Schaffer, F. (2005) Suppression of inflammatory and fibrotic responses in allergic inflammation by the amniotic membrane stromal matrix. *Clin Exp Allergy, 35*, 941-8.

[171] Hao, Y., Ma, D. H., Hwang, D. G., Kim, W. S. & Zhang, F. (2000) Identification of antiangiogenic and antiinflammatory proteins in human amniotic membrane. *Cornea, 19*, 348-52.

[172] Solomon, A., Rosenblatt, M., Monroy, D., Ji, Z., Pflugfelder, S. C. & Tseng, S. C. (2001) Suppression of interleukin 1alpha and interleukin 1beta in human limbal epithelial cells cultured on the amniotic membrane stromal matrix. *Br J Ophthalmol, 85*, 444-9.

[173] Kamiya, K., Wang, M., Uchida, S., Amano, S., Oshika, T., Sakuragawa, N. & Hori, J. (2005) Topical application of culture supernatant from human amniotic epithelial cells suppresses inflammatory reactions in cornea. *Exp Eye Res, 80*, 671-9.

[174] Li, W., He, H., Kawakita, T., Espana, E. M. & Tseng, S. C. (2006) Amniotic membrane induces apoptosis of interferon-gamma activated macrophages in vitro. *Exp Eye Res, 82*, 282-92.

[175] Lee, P., Wang, C. C. & Adamis, A. P. (1998) Ocular neovascularization: an epidemiologic review. *Surv Ophthalmol, 43*, 245-69.

[176] Kobayashi, N., Kabuyama, Y., Sasaki, S., Kato, K. & Homma, Y. (2002) Suppression of corneal neovascularization by culture supernatant of human amniotic cells. *Cornea, 21*, 62-7.

[177] Shao, C., Sima, J., Zhang, S. X., Jin, J., Reinach, P., Wang, Z. & Ma, J. X. (2004) Suppression of corneal neovascularization by PEDF release from human amniotic membranes. *Invest Ophthalmol Vis Sci, 45*, 1758-62.

[178] Jiang, A., Li, C., Gao, Y., Zhang, M., Hu, J., Kuang, W., Hao, S., Yang, W., Xu, C., Gao, G., Wang, Z. & Liu, Z. (2006) In vivo and in vitro inhibitory effect of amniotic extraction on neovascularization. *Cornea, 25*, S36-40.

[179] Koizumi, N. J., Inatomi, T. J., Sotozono, C. J., Fullwood, N. J., Quantock, A. J. & Kinoshita, S. (2000) Growth factor mRNA and protein in preserved human amniotic membrane. *Curr Eye Res, 20*, 173-7.

[180] Kjaergaard, N., Hein, M., Hyttel, L., Helmig, R. B., Schonheyder, H. C., Uldbjerg, N. & Madsen, H. (2001) Antibacterial properties of human amnion and chorion in vitro. *Eur J Obstet Gynecol Reprod Biol, 94*, 224-9.

[181] Rubin, L. R. & Bongiovi, J., Jr. (1971) Human skin--antibacterial in vitro? *J Surg Res, 11*, 321-4.

[182] Galask, R. P. & Snyder, I. S. (1970) Antimicrobial factors in amniotic fluid. *Am J Obstet Gynecol, 106*, 59-65.

[183] Otsuki, K., Yoda, A., Saito, H., Mitsuhashi, Y., Toma, Y., Shimizu, Y. & Yanaihara, T. (1999) Amniotic fluid lactoferrin in intrauterine infection. *Placenta, 20*, 175-9.

[184] Talmi, Y. P., Sigler, L., Inge, E., Finkelstein, Y. & Zohar, Y. (1991) Antibacterial properties of human amniotic membranes. *Placenta, 12*, 285-8.

[185] Kjaergaard, N., Helmig, R. B., Schonheyder, H. C., Uldbjerg, N., Hansen, E. S. & Madsen, H. (1999) Chorioamniotic membranes constitute a competent barrier to group b streptococcus in vitro. *Eur J Obstet Gynecol Reprod Biol, 83*, 165-9.

Reviewed by:

Gian Paolo Bagnara, Department of Histology, Embryology and Applied Biology, University of Bologna, Italy (bagnara@alma.unibo.it)

Giacomo Lanzoni, Department of Histology, Embryology and Applied Biology, University of Bologna, Italy (giacomo.lanzoni@unibo.it)

Thomas John, MD, Clinical Associate Professor, Loyola University at Chicago, Maywood, IL, USA and in private practice in Tinley Park and Oak Lawn, IL,USA (tjcornea@gmail.com)

In: Human Placenta: Structure and Development... ISBN: 978-1-60876-457-0
Editors: E. Berven, et al. pp. 49-77 © 2010 Nova Science Publishers, Inc.

Chapter II

Dynamic Role of Trophoblast in Human Placental Development

Dong-Hyun Cha[1] and Gi Jin Kim[2]

[1]Department of Obstetrics and Gynecology, CHA General Hospital, CHA University, Seoul, Korea.

[2]Department of Biomedical Science CHA University, Seoul, Korea.

The placenta, which is a temporary organ derived from the fetus, is removed after delivery. This organ is critical to support fetus development via optimal regulation between mother and fetus. The placenta includes different cell types: amnion, trophoblast, decidual cells, Hofbauer cells, endothelium, and mesenchymal cells. Among these cell types, the trophoblast is one of the earliest to differentiate and shows an extensive proliferation or/and differentiation up to the formation of the normal placenta as a major cell population. The characterization of the trophoblast shows dynamic changes according to placental development during pregnancy. This brief review outlines the development of the trophoblast and its function in the placenta during pregnancy. We review how the trophoblast can play a role in developmental processes under various environment factors and link this function to gynecological diseases. Finally, we introduce the latest research in trophoblast differentiation and the therapeutic potential of trophoblast stem cells for obstetrical and gynecological diseases.

Introduction

The root of life begins at fertilization through sequences of coordinated events when a male gamete (sperm) and a female gamete (oocyte) form a single cell (zygote). Repeated mitotic divisions of the zygote rapidly form blastocysts, consisting of two primary cell types including the inner cell mass known as the 'embryoblast" and the trophectoderm also known as the "trophoblast" [1]. The trophoblast later forms the placenta (Figure 1). Implantation of the blastocyst into the endometrium of the maternal uterus is completed by the end of the second week after fertilization [2]. This implantation is mediated by invasion of the differentiated trophoblast (e.g. syncytiotrophoblast) from the trophectoderm. Although the trophectoderm originated from the fetus, it is never incorporated into the cells of the mother's body. In addition to this, the trophoblast is one of the earliest cell types to differentiate and displays an extensive proliferation or/and differentiation up to the formation of the normal placenta as a major cell population [1, 3].

During pregnancy, the unique role of the trophoblast is to invasion, eroding, and metastasizing in the placenta as well as to ensure appropriate bidirectional nutrient or waste flow required for growth and maturation of the embryo. The syncytiotrophoblast, localized in the outer-line of placental villi, is particularly important to express essential factors (e.g. growth factors, hormones, enzymes and so on) at the correct time and the right location to facilitate optimal fetal development [3]. The word 'trophoblast' is derived from tropho which means "to feed" and blastos which means "germinator". According to placental development during pregnancy, the characterizations of trophoblasts show dynamic changes through differentiation under several environmental factors in the extracellular matrix and maternal blood of the placenta and uterus. Finally, the trophoblasts develop into a large part of the placenta, which support fetal development via the several regulation factors such as growth factors, hormones, cytokines, and so on between mother and fetus during pregnancy [4]. The dysfunction of the trophoblast during pregnancy can result in several gynecological diseases including congenital malformation in neonatal medicine. Therefore, trophoblasts act as a conclusive factor in placental and fetal development.

This brief review outlines the development of the trophoblast and its function in the placenta during pregnancy. We also review how the trophoblast can play a role in developmental processes under various environment factors and links this function to gynecological diseases. Finally, we introduce the latest research in trophoblast differentiation and the therapeutic potential of trophoblast stem cells in obstetrical and gynecological diseases.

I. Trophoblast Development during Pregnancy

Implantation of the blastocyst into the maternal endometrium, mediated by well-differentiated primary cells of the placenta known as trophoblasts, grow in an invasive and destructive fashion similar to tumor cells [5,6]. However, these cells are limited and regulated in space and time. The differentiation of trophoblasts derived from the outer layer of the blastocyst after fertilization rapidly progress through a complex network of signaling molecules that mediate cell-to-cell and cell-to-extracellular matrix communications. This finally culminates in the controlled invasion of the trophoblast and induced successful implantation [7,8]. After implantation, trophoblast cells proliferate and differentiate along two lineages for villous and extravillous trophoblast. Generally, villous cytotrophoblast cells form the outer epithelial layer of the chorionic villi as well as multinucleated syncytiotrophoblasts via cell fusion. Their major function is to facilitate the exchange of fetal and maternal metabolites including hormones, nutrients, wastes, and gas. Otherwise, extravillous trophoblast cells, which have a potential for invasion, migrate into the decidua and the basal matrix on the maternal endometrium [9]. These cells finally induce remodeling of uterine arteries in the endometrium. Several substances are metabolized and these metabolic products are released into maternal and fetal circulations. [10]

During the trophoblast differentiation, this outer layer is divided into two different cell types such as cytotrophoblast and syncytiotrophoblast when they begin differentiation. The cytotrophoblast as a single nucleate cell is located in the inner layer of the trophectoderm and exerts a strong proliferative activity thereby classifying it as a trophoblast stem cell [11-13]. These cells also migrate into the syncytiotrophoblast to increase the population of finally differentiated syncytiotrophoblasts through fusion and losing of their cell membrane. Otherwise, the syncytiotrophoblast known as syncytium is a mutilnucleate cell, which covers the surface of the placental villi and forms as a result of the differentiated trophoblast via multiple process including fusion of the between underlying cytotrophoblasts during placental developmnet. The syncytiotrophoblast grows into the endometrial stroma and plays a role as a barrier function of the placenta as well as produces several hormones. The syncytiotrophoblast secretes human chorionic gonadotrophin (hCG) to maintain the hormonal activity of the corpus luteum, which secretes estrogen and progesterone to sustain the pregnancy in the ovary [14]. The expression of hCG secreted by syncytiotrophoblasts at the end of the second week can be detected using a positive pregnancy test. Most of the early pregnancy factors are immunosuppressant proteins and are secreted into the maternal serum by the syncytiotrophoblast within 24 hours to 49 hours after fertilization [15].

Most cellular and syncytial trophoblasts from previllous stages of placentation are consumed for the development of the placental villi. It forms the villous cytotrophoblast and the villous syncytiotrophoblast. The remaining trophoblasts that are unconsumed for villous formation are referred to as extravillous trophoblasts. These form the basic materials for the development of all nonvillous portions of the placenta [3]. They are located on the resting on the basal lamina of villi, cell columns, cell islands, chorionic plates and smooth chorion; the extravillous trophoblasts are distinguished markedly in their shape and staining patterns. The nonvillous trophoblast stem cells differentiate into villous syncytiotrophoblast or extravillous trophoblasts depending on the communication with maternal blood or the maternal extracellular matrix as the main environmental factors [16]. The proliferative activities of extravillous trophoblasts increase when they are in closer proximity to the basal lamina of the neighboring fetal stroma of anchoring villous. The proliferation markers (e.g. PCNA, Ki-67) recognize extravillous trophoblasts, which show proliferative phenotypes in the underlying basal lamina. Non-proliferative extravillous trophoblasts, which are differentiated to a greater extent, are located on the distal part of placental villi derived from the nearest proliferative center by migration or invasion into the myometrium. Some extravillous trophoblasts differentiate into the invasive extravillous trophoblast through invasion into the maternal myometrium; finally, they divided into the endovascular trophoblasts and multinuclated trophoblasts according to contact with maternal blood or blood vessels (Figure 2). This differentiational regulation is known to be accomplished by different factors including cytokines and hormones, which are produced by both fetal as well as maternal tissues i.e., placenta and uterus, respectively [16, 17]. Growth factors such as EGF, IGF-2, and HGF are known to influence trophoblast migration, while cytokines such as leptin and M-CSF are known to regulate trophoblast proliferation, and leukemia inhibitory factor (LIF) is a representative factor for trophoblast invasion [18-20]. Each factor utilizes at least one pathway for the intracellular signaling within trophoblast differentiation and their invasion in several functions, essential regulating factors in this process still not fully understood. The invasive activity of extravillous trophoblasts into the maternal uterine wall is controlled by tight regulation via several cytokines and hormones at the correct time and designated space. The extravillous trophoblasts are similar to cancer cells in that they migrate and invade the uterus and its vasculatures thatprovide a vital link between the mother and the developing fetus through complex endocrine, paracrine and autocrine means [17; 21]. The extravillous trophoblast in particular, secretes large amounts of highly heterogeneous extracellular matrix proteins along their invasion routes. The extracellular matrix proteins secreted from invading extravillous trophoblast are regulated by extracellular matrix receptors (Integrins); other cell adhesion molecules and gap junction molecules exist on the surface of the maternal myometrium and the extravillous trophoblast. When extravillous trophoblasts invade the myometrium, the degradation of the endometrial extracellular matrix is regulated by activities of various proteinases (matrix metalloproteinsase, MMPs), plasminogen activators and tissue inhibitors (TIMPs) [19; 22]. Moreover, the invasion of extravillous trophoblasts is repressed by the products of the *KiSS-1* gene (kisspeptins), which is a melanoma metastasis suppressor gene, via binding to the G protein-coupled receptor KiSS-1R as well as the Janus kinase-signal transducers and activators of transcription (Jak-Stat) and the receptor-associated tyrosine kinase-mitogen-activated protein kinase (RTK-MAPK) pathways [23-25]. The trophoblast is capable of differentiating towards specific cell types and this is a useful tool for the study of the mechanism of differentiation of trophoblasts during placental development.

Several phenotypes for trophoblast development are regulated by the rapid trophoblast turnover and its dynamics. In the first trimester of pregnancy, the cytotrophoblast proliferative activity is high, but this is significantly decreased in the third trimester of pregnancy. Because most of the increased cytotrophoblasts are subsequently incorporated into the syncytiotrophoblast by cell fusion, a large proportion of syncyial nuclei are subsequently extruded by apoptosis, and thus the number and function of syncytiotrophoblasts are regulated and maintained [26]. Apoptosis of syncytiotrophoblast knotting, known as syncytial knotting, is one of the phenotypes for trophoblast degeneration and results in knot-like structures showing on smooth surfaces of developing microvilli [27]. The shedding of syncytial knotting from microvilli into the maternal circulation provides a means of analyzing the genetic information of the fetus. Syncytial knotting show highly condensed chromatin and an increase in the population within the placental villi Increased abnormal syncytial knotting (trophoblastic apoptosis) causes gynecological diseases through the inhibition or decreasing of the function and development of trophoblasts in the placenta. Trophoblastic apoptosis is resistant to Fas-mediated apoptosis because trophoblasts normally express high levels of FasL but lower levels of Fas. Trophoblastic apoptosis mediated Fas signaling is promoted by IFN-gamma and TNF-alpha, whereas their resistance is increased by activation of FLICE-like inhibitory protein (FLIP), a downstream inhibitor of Fas apoptotic signaling through IL-10 cytokine treatment [28, 29]

Thus, the balance between proliferation and apoptosis of trophoblasts is physiologically important for the processes of trophoblast differentiation and placental development. Excessive or pathological apoptosis of trophoblasts leads to poor placental development and fetal growth retardation and is associated with gynecological diseases.

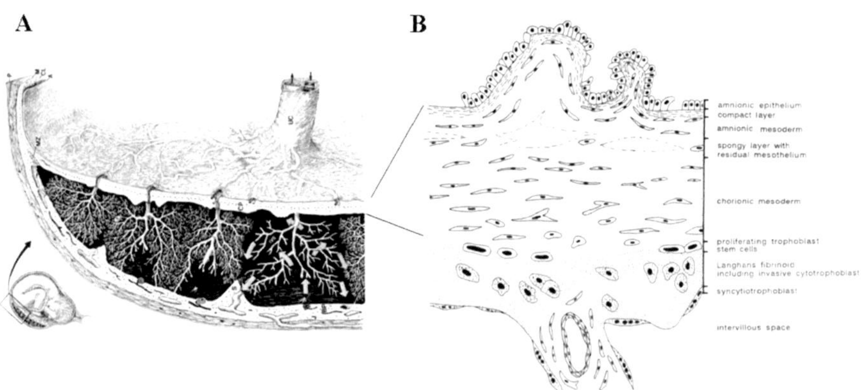

Figure 1. The structure of human placenta. (A) Placenta is composed of the chorionic plate (CP), the intervillous space (IVS), and the basal plate (BP). Each abbreviate means the following; P=perimetrium, M=myometirum, Cl=chorion leave, A= amnion, MZ=marginal zone between placenta and fetal menbranes, UC=umbilical cord, S=placental septum. (B) Several types of cells located on the fetal menbranes including anchoring villi. (Adapted from Benirschke K; Kaufmann P. Pathology of the Human Placenta, 4th ed. New York, 2000).

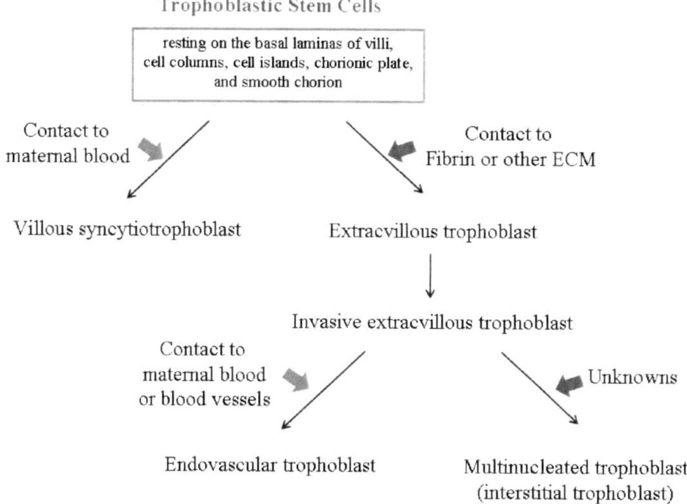

Figure 2. In vivo trophoblast differentiation depend on the environmental factors (modified by Benirschke K; Kaufmann P. Pathology of the Human Placenta, 4th ed. New York, 2000).

II. Correlation between Gene Expression and Trophoblast Differentiation

Communication between the maternal endometrium and trophoblast during implantation is important in trophoblast differentiation for successful placental development. Succesful trophoblast differentiation is dependent on expression of developmental regulatory genes; further differentiation leading to embryonic implantation on the endometrium of the uterus requires various factors existing in the microenvironment [30]. Recently, Robert et al demonstrated the networking from early trophectoderm to invasive extravillous cytotrophoblasts between the trophoblast differentiation-regulated factors using *in vitro* stem cell culture system (Figure 3) [31]. The balance of Oct-4 expression role as a key factor for the decision of cell fate between inner cell mass (ICM) and trophectoderm in the early morula stage, the alteration of Cdx2, Gcm1, Id2, Mash2, and MMP9 and cytokine treatment (e.g. BMP4, bFGF, and bHLH) were shown to be sequentially involved in trophoblast differentiation [32]. Moreover, early trophoblast proliferation is dependent on the gap junction proteins (e.g. Cx31) and growth factors (e.g. FGF, Nodal). These cascade steps induce the changes in morphology and function of trophoblasts as well as trophoblast differentiation through cell fusion of cytotrophoblasts [31, 33, 34].

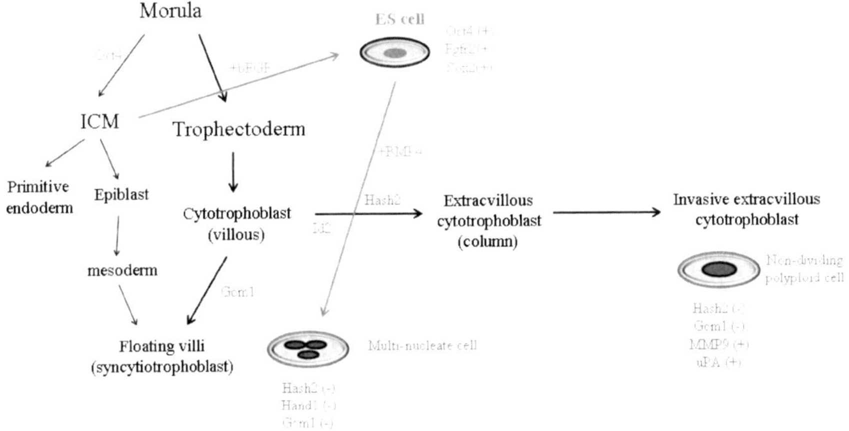

Figure 3. In vitro trophoblast differentiation from the trophectoderm of Morular stage using several cytokines (modified by Roberts RM and their colleagues; Reprod Biol Endocrinol. 2004).

During trophoblast differentiation, the trophoblast cell lineage divides into two major lineages, an "invasive trophoblast" cell subtype, and a "transport trophoblast" cell subtype. Although the mechanism and related factors for trophoblast differentiation are still not fully understood, many studies have focused on extravillous trophoblast differentiation because trophoblast differentiation is mediated through multiple molecules and signaling cascades via interaction between invaded trophoblasts and various emanating factors from the maternal endometrium [4, 11]. Extravillous trophoblast differentiation is regulated by numerous growth factors, extracellular matrix proteins and adhesion molecules expressed at the fetal-maternal interface. These regulatory molecules regulate cell invasion by modulating the activities of matrix-degrading proteases (e.g. MMPs, inhibitors) and adhesion molecules (e.g. integrins, cadherins, connexins) on the extracellular matrix [3; 35]. In addition to this, numerous signaling cascades/proteins including GTPases, RhoA, protein kinases ROCK, ERK1, ERK2, FAK, PI3K, Akt/protein kinase B, homeobox genes (e.g. DLX4, HB24, MSX2 and MOX2) and mTOR as well as TGF-beta-dependent SMAD factors has been known to be involved in trophoblast differentiation [36, 37].

Among these regulatory or signaling factors, transforming growth factor beta (TGF-beta) has been shown to be a multifunctional cytokine required for embryonic development as well as regulation of trophoblast behavior [38]. TGF-beta cytokines and their signaling pathway are well known in the regulation of apoptosis, invasion and differentiation of extravillous trophoblasts. Recent studies report that PL74/gdf15/MIC-1, PL48, a new serine-threonine protein kinase, serum and glucocorticoid-induced kinase, PBK-1, a tunicamycin-responsive gene, a cathepsin D-like gene (DAP-1), hypoxia- regulated genes HRF-1,2,6,8 and HIF-1alpha, HIF-1beta, as well as hEPAS-1 are involved in the tight control of TGF-beta signaling, thereby regulating apoptosis and differentiation of extravillous trophoblasts [21, 39, 40]. Also, TGF-beta signaling has multiple functions in the regulation of trophoblast differentiation as well as trophoblast invasion through the repression of production of the proenzyme MMP-9 and the upregulation of expression of epithelial-cadherin and beta-catenin [41]. Physiological factors including exchange of oxygen tension under hypoxic environments is essential for the formation of the fetal-maternal interface. Consequently embryonic development in early pregnancy prevents trophoblast differentiation and promotes trophoblast proliferation. Un-regulated hypoxia-inducible factor-1 (HIF-1), a master regulator of oxygen homeostasis, controls the expression of TGF-beta 3 and acts as an inhibitor of extravillous trophoblast differentiation [42]. Hypoxia also regulates cell fate by triggering the exit from the cell cycle and subsequent differentiation of trophoblasts.

In the case of cytotrophoblasts, various chemokine receptors that can bind ligands expressed at locations on the near trophoblasts could be implicated. The chemokine, syncytin, which is a cell fusion-inducing gene, ERV-3 gene, which is cloned from term placenta, and Endoglin, PlGF, TGF-beta3, IGF-II, IGFBP-1, as well as a placental IGFBP protease have all been reported to associate in the regulation ofproliferation, differentiation and migration of cytotrophoblasts [37, 43]. Furthermore, differentiation through communication between trophoblasts process via connexin expression and gap junctional intercellular communication (GJIC) on the surface of trophoblasts. The expression and interaction of connexins is important in regulating trophoblastic differentiation. Among these connexins, the expression of Cx31 and Cx40 plays a critical role in the switch from a proliferative to an invasive phenotype of trophoblastic cells invading the endometrium. Also, the expression of Cx43 allows the proliferation of trophoblasts and GJIC required for the fusion process of cytotrophoblastic cells, leading to the formation of the syncytiotrophoblast which is the site of numerous placental functions [16, 44].

Taken together, cascades for trophoblast differentiation progress dynamically via the harmony infused by a multiplicity of factors including transcription factors, growth factors, cytokines, chemokines, adhesion molecules, and microenvironment factors (e.g. hypoxia) as well as cell-to-cell communication through connexins. This processing is tightly regulated by the correct time and designated space from the blastocyst stage until placental development.

III. Correlation between Trophoblast Dysfunction and Obstetrical/ Gynecological Diseases

This section summarized our current understanding of the mechanism of preeclampsia and intrauterine growth restriction (IUGR), with an emphasis on the recently characterized endothelial dysfunction via circulating anti-angiogenic proteins and the inadequacy of trophoblast invasion among various gynecological diseases. It is well known that dilation of spiral arteries in the maternal myometrium is necessary to establish successful placentation and to increase the blood supply to the developing fetus [45, 46]. This physiological modification is thought to be brought about by the invasion of cytotrophoblasts into the spiral artery vessel wall. The trophoblastic invasion is a key process during placentation, and a process that allows an adequate vascular connection between the intervillous space and the maternal blood flow. Although many studies on the mechanisms that control human trophoblast invasion in between implantation and normal placentation have been attempted, this process is still poorly understood due to difficulties in obtaining correct samples from placental bed biopsies. These biopsies are a useful source for the study of trophoblast invasion into the spiral artery vessel wall in substance [46].

The invasion of extravillous trophoblasts into spiral arteries in maternal decidual tissues and myometrium, is similar to tumor invasion, but trophoblast invasion is limited in the first trimester of pregnancy and on the proximal third of the myometrium. It is also known to be subject to various influences such as genetic, microenvironment, and immunologic factors. Extravillous cytotrophoblasts from anchoring villi migrate in a retrograde direction along the spiral arteries, endovascular trophoblasts, transforming them into large diameter conduit vessels of low resistance through the decidual segments of spiral arteries and the myometrial segments [47]. Therefore, the dysfunction or abnormal invasion of extravillous cytotrophoblasts due to defects in the trophoblastic differentiating pathways including endovascular, interstitial and chorionic villous could be induced in severe dysfunction of the endothelium in the networking of complicated vessels in placenta, resulting in the trigger of pathogenesis of early-onset gynecology diseases such as intra-uterine growth restriction (IUGR), pre-eclampsia and etc (Figure 4). The erosion of defective endovascular trophoblast could lead to failures of dilation in the spiral arteriole at the placental bed of the maternal myometrium as an early implantated site. Defective invasion of interstitial extravillous trophoblasts at the erosion of the distal spiral arteriole can delay the development of villi as well as induce problems of local angiogenic and systemic vascular adaptation to improve uterine blood flow [48, 49]. Lowering of blood pressure and prevention of eclampsia are indicated in severe preeclampsia.

The risk factors causing dysfunction of endothelial cells by inadequate invasive activities of endovascular and interstitial trophoblasts are generally closely associated with angiogenic factors (e.g. placental growth factor, PlGF, vascular endothelial growth factor, VEGF, soluble VEGF receptor-1, sVEGFR-1 and soluble endoglin) and matrix-degrading proteases such as MMPs and inhibitors, which control invasion of trophoblast [50]. VEGF and their receptors are the best-characterized endothelial-specific growth factors that increase vascular permeability and angiogenesis as well as cytokines having multiple biological functions in the vascular development. The family of VEGF-related molecules comprise of seven sub-families including VEGF, placenta growth factor (PLGF), and VEGF-B, -C, -D, -E, and –F. The biological functions of each family are mediated by the different receptors such as VEGFR-1/Flt-1, VEGFR-2/Flk-1, VEGFR-3/Flt-4, co-receptors of neuropilin (NRP) and heparan sulfate proteoglycans (HSPGs) [51, 52]. These factors regulate exposure to hypoxic conditions, which is similar to inducing angiogenesis of cancer cells for carcinogenesis.

Hypoxia is a responsible factor for physiologic placental development as well as angiogenesis. Generally, hypoxia inducible factor 1a (HIF-1a) is stable and initiates gene transcription under hypoxia, whereas it interaction with the von Hippel-Lindau tumor suppressor protein (VHL) lead to rapid degradation of them in normoxia. It is regulated by temporal and spatial changes in expression and association of molecules forming the multi-protein VHLCBC complex. So, HIF-1a, which expressed in cytotrophoblasts in the early plaentation, mediates placental morphogenesis, angiogenesis, and cell fate decisions, demonstrating that O2 tension is a critical regulator of trophoblast lineage determination [53, 54]. These hypoxic condition increases VEGF and sVEGFR-1 expressions through induction of oxidative stress of trophoblasts via increased lipid peroxide production in the early placental development. The dysregulation of the PlGF/VEGF axis in the maternal circulation derived from trophoblasts is reversed except the expression of endoglin when trophoblasts were exposed to hypoxic condition (Figure 5) [50, 55-58]. Also, the cascades for overproduction of VEGF family factors and sVEGFR-1 by hypoxia, overproduction of hypoxic villous trophoblasts causing maternal free VEGF depletion, and low circulating level of free PlGF are progressing [59]. So, these unbalanced circulating angiogenic proteins are involved in the function of trophoblasts and finally results in several gynecological diseases.

IUGR and pre-eclampsia are as representative of the main gynecological diseases that involve the dysfunction of endothelium via insufficiency of trophoblasts. These are a significant cause of infant mortality and morbidity through the development of placental insufficiency [60, 61]. The dysfunction of endothelial cells causes maternal hypertension, edema, and proteinuria, with direct or indirect influence on arterial permeability in pre-eclampsia. The phenotypes for pre-eclampsia are diagnosed at the second trimester during the pregnancy. Until now, numerous studies attempting to elucidate the exact etiopathogenesis of this complex multifactorial disease, prediction or prevention methods of preeclampsia have been conducted. However, the etiologies for pre-eclmapsia and IUGR are still unknown and biomakers for diagnostic purposes are insufficient in early pregnancy. Therefore, many scientists have focused on the correlation between endothelial dysfunction and trophoblast invasion in the remodeling of arteries to develop biomarkers that could be useful in the detection of these phenotypes in early pregnancy. As the described above, the expression levels for angiogenic factors including VEGF, PlGF, their receptors, and endoglin in maternal blood are useful makers in the diagnosis of gynecological diseases such as pre-eclampsia and IUGR.

In addition to this, the factors for adhesion, detachment from the extracellular matrix (ECM), invasion of the ECM and maternal vessels by proteolysis via trophoblast targeting have been reported to be closely associated with pre-eclampsia and IUGR [62-64]. Particularly, the complicated repertoire of adhesion molecules including intercellular adhesion molecule-1 (ICAM-1), fibronectin and integrin alpha5, plasminogen activator inhibitor (PAI)-1, melanoma cell adhesion molecule (Mel-CAM), Mucin I (MUC1), urokinase-type plasminogen activator (uPA), and various proteinases could regulate the degradation of the endometrial extracellular matrix such as gelatinase A and B (MMP-2 and MMP-9), decorin (a proteoglycan in the ECM) [65-67]. These could also inhibit the tissue inhibitor of matrix metalloprotease 1 (TIMP-1) and plasminogen activator inhibitor (PAI-1). Thus these molecules were studied for the evaluation of the activity for trophoblast invasion in pre-eclampsia. In case of integrins, they participate in cell-cell adhesion as well as in adhesion between cells and components of the extracellular matrix [16]. Their expressional changes are synchronized with trophoblast attachment. For example, the expression of integrins alpha5beta3, alpha4beta1, alpha6beta1, and alpha7beta1 is related to the stages of bryo-endometrium interactions; otherwise, the cascade patterns in the stages of the embryonic invasion into the deciduas relates as follows: integrins alpha6beta4→alpha5beta1→alpha1beta1 →alpha4beta1. Therefore, switching of integrin expression patterns is associated with several diseases, including preeclampsia, intrauterine growth retardation caused by vascular problems [68-70].

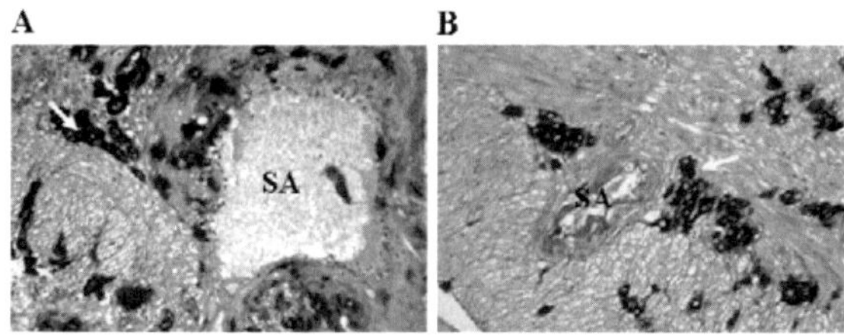

Figure 4. Comparison of the dilation of spiral arteries in placental bed biopsy between normal (A) and pre-eclamptic placenta (B) using cytokeratin 7 and PAS staining. SA means spiral arteries, yellow arrow means interstitial trophoblast, red arrow means endovascular trophoblast in the spiral arteries.

Phosphorylation of trophoblast invasion-regulated signaling, e.g. phosphorylation of mitogen-activated protein kinase (MAPK), focal adhesion kinase (FAK) and MAPK (ERK-1 and ERK-2) leads to increased trophoblastic invasion [71- 73]. Therefore, these biomarkers could be used as useful diagnosis markers for pre-eclmapsia or IUGR. Dipeptidyl peptidase IV

(DPPIV), carboxypeptidase-M (CP-M), and novel membrane-bound cell surface peptidase (laeverin), which are cell surface peptidases, have been reported to associate with an increased trophoblastic invasion through the interaction of RANTES, a substrate of DPPIV and its receptor, CCR1 [74-76].

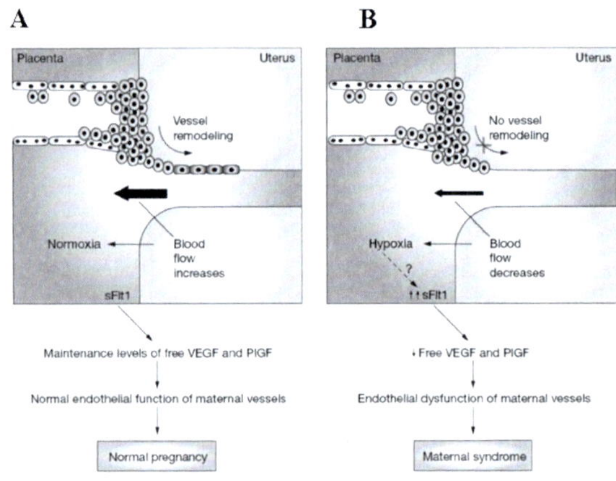

Figure 5. Correlation between the vessel remodeling by trophoblast invasion and the expression of angiogenic factors in normal placenta (A) and pre-eclamptic placenta (B) under hypoxic condition. (modified by Noris M and their colleagues; Nat Clin Pract Nephrol. 2005).

Recently, many scientists have reported genes expression profiling associated with widespread endothelial dysfunction in pre-eclampsia and several functional modules associated with either invasive or noninvasive trophoblast phenotype using Gene Chip micro arrays. The selected genes including ECGF1, JAG1, Palladin, COL18A1, TNFSF12, VEGF, ANPEP, PDGFRA, SERPIN12, EPAS1, FLT1, heme oxygenase-1 (HO-1), nuclear hormone receptor peroxisome proliferator activated receptor (PPAR) gamma, SIGLE10 and ANG4 were evaluated. From the gene profiling study, new biomarkers could be developed for the diagnosis and the better understanding of the pathophysiological characters of pre-eclampsia [77-79].

Finally, the invasion of trophoblasts is also mediated by the physiologic systems that appear to have evolved to sustain the metabolic regulation via peroxisome proliferator-activated receptors (PPARs). PPAR-gamma binds excessive oxidized LDLs, resulting in the modulation of trophoblastic invasion in the early first trimester. Therefore, the inadequate regulation of the PPAR system influences the trophoblastic invasion through the dysregulation of metabolism, inflammation and angiogenesis [78, 80]. Also, many inflammatory cytokines and immune factors including those based on maternal immunity as well as the unique immune environment of the placental bed regulate the invasive activity of trophoblasts. Immune cells such as decidual natural killer (NK) cells and macrophages supply factors necessary for arterial modification of the maternal-fetal interface through the secretion of inflammatory cytokines, chemokines, angiogeneic factors and proteinases in the first trimester [81-83]. A system of immune tolerance present between maternal and fetal interface. Among these system affect by several factors, the increased expression of IL-2, IL-4, IL-6, IL-10, IFN-γ and TNF-α secreted from type I and II of helper T (Th1 and 2) cells derived from the maternal myometrium attack the trophoblastic invasion derived from the fetus. Also, the expression of Toll-like receptors (TLRs) on the trophoblast control the decidualization when they contact to the decidual layer and the inhibition of endovascular invasion by activated macrophage-induced apoptosis of trophoblast resulting happened the inadequacy trophoblast invasion on the placental bed [84, 85;. Otherwise, the combination of maternal killer-immunoglobulin-like receptors (KIR) on NK cells fetal HLA-C, which affects the balance between inhibition and activation signals of NK cells, regulatory CD8(+) T cells (cytotoxic T cells), and regulatory NK cells, may play very important roles in the induction of MHC class I-specific tolerance [86, 87]. Interestingly, trophoblastic cells are unique because they are one of the few mammalian cell types that do not express major histocompatibility complex (MHC) class II antigens. The extravillous trophoblast expresses HLA-G among the MHC antigens, which is different to embryoblast-derived cells. The expressed of HLA-G act to suppress immunological of NK cells and controls trophoblast invasion [88, 89].

Otherwise, the excessive invasion of trophoblasts into the maternal myometirum causes gestational trophoblastic diseases (GTDs), which represent a unique group of lesions because they are derived from the fetus and not from the mother. Gestational trophoblastic diseases result from an abnormal proliferation of differentiated types of trophoblasts. Among the various GTDs, choriocarcinoma has great propensities of vascular invasion as well as metastases to the lung and the brain. These frequencies of choriocarcinoma are relative to its various precursors such as hydatidiform mole, ectopic pregnancy and habitual abortions and the levels of hCG produced by differentiated syncytotrophoblast [90]. Also, the regulation of excessive invasions of trophoblasts are associated with the above mentioned factors, which are growth factors, cytokines, proteinases, adhesion molecules, and various signaling pathways via Stat3 [75, 91].

Therefore, trophoblast invasion, which is a unique capability, is similar to tumor development although it is temporally and locally controlled in contrast to unlimited tumor invasion. It is tightly controlled by positive or negative regulation through communications between trophoblast and a number of other factors during early pregnancy. However, the suppression of the development of villi as well as the dilation of endothelial cells in the placenta induces gynecological diseases such as pre-eclampsia, IUGR, and gestational trophoblastic neoplasia (GTN).

IV. The Latest Research in Trophoblasts and the Therapeutic Potential of Trophoblast Stem Cells in Obstetrical and Gynecological Diseases

Here, we introduce the latest research in characterization of trophoblast stem cells and focus on the possibility of their application in obstetrical and gynecology diseases. Trophoblast research over the past decades has underlined striking similarities between proliferative, migratory and invasive properties of placental cells and those of cancer cells because of the unique characteristics of trophoblasts such as aneuplod by cell fusion and invasion in normal development. Since various trophoblast-specific transcriptions have been related to placental diseases, many studies on trophoblasts focused on the alteration of gene expression based on differentiation in early stages of development [60]. Recently, trophoendodermal stem cells as known to trophoblast stem cells have been deemed a useful material for the study of the mechanism as well as gene profiling of trophoblast differentiation [13, 92, 93]. Similar to embryonic stem cells, trophoblast stem cells have the potential for self-renewal and differentiation into various types of trophoblasts (e.g. syntithiotrophoblast, interstitial trophoblast, endovascular trophoblasts, etc). They can spontaneously differentiate into several types of trophoblasts from the trophectoderm of blastocysts and express cytokeratin 7 and HLA-G (Figure 6). Their stemness is maintained and regulated by stimulation of FGF4, heparin and fibroblast-conditioned medium, whereas differentiation and/or maintenance of the differentiated derivatives are dependent on key transcription factors such as Oct4, Nanog, CDX2, ATP1B3, SFN, Ets2, IPL, and Hand1 and signaling pathway (e.g. Wnt, MAPK, TGF-β, NOTCH, and integrin-mediated cell adhesion) [32, 94, 95]. The epigenetic regulation of the POU-family transcription factor, Oct3/4 genes between embryonic stem and trophoblast stem cells are different; the promoter region of the Oct4 gene is hypomethylated in embryonic stem cells (ES cells), but is hypermethylated in trophoblast stem (TS) cells, in which the Oct4 gene is repressed [93]. Also, the alterations of Oct4-dependent genes are regulated directly by Oct4 either positively (e.g. ZFP42, LEFTY1, LEFTY2, DPPA4, THY1, FLJ10884, and TDGF1) or negatively (e.g. EOMES, BMP4, fibroblast growth factor 8 (FGF8), DKK1, HLX1, GATA2, GATA6, ID2, and DLX5) decide the cell fate of trophoblast stem cells through various differentiation steps [96]. The epigenetic regulation of Nanog genes between embryonic stem and trophoblast stem cells is associated with the differentially methylated region (T-DMR) in the Nanog up-stream region. The expression of the Nanog gene is hypomethylated in embryonic stem cells, but is hypermethylated in trophoblast stem cells, in which the Nanog gene is repressed through DNA methylation and histone modifications of Nanog gene [95]. Also, the overexpression of Caudal-related homeobox 2 (Cdx2), which is sufficient to generate proper trophoblast stem cells, decides the fate of cells between the inner cell mass and trophectoderm in the early blastocyst. These Cdx2 expressions are dispensable for trophectoderm differentiation induced by Oct3/4 repression but essential for TS cell self-renewal [97]. Therefore, these balanced regulations of various genes, which are expressed in the early stage of blastocysts trigger the cascade of differentiation in trophoblast stem cells. Thus, trophoblast stem cells have important clinical and basic experimental potential and consequently can be used as a useful in vitro model for the study of embyogenesis in early pregnancy [98]. The role of trophoblast cells in regulation of trophoblast differentiation, invasion, and gynecological diseases such as pre-eclampsia, IUGR as well as infertility mechanisms depends on the implantation condition.

Takahashi and their colleagues reported the therapeutic effect of trophoblasts in suppressing cytokine signaling 3 (SOCS3), which is a negative regulator of cytokine signaling-deficient mice using trophoblast stem cells. Harun et al. reported that cytotrophoblast stem cells derived from human embryonic stem cells showed the mimic phenotype similar to the invasive implantation events. Thus the clinical applications of trophoblast stem cells in various gynecological diseases including vessel remodeling, abnormal invasion, and immune rejection [99, 100] are continuously being attempted. Although there are many changes to overcome in applying cell therapy using trophoblast stem cells, if the basic research for the establishment and the characterization of trophoblast stem cells including pre-clinical data is undergone, this allows for the potential for new therapies in reproductive medicine in the future.

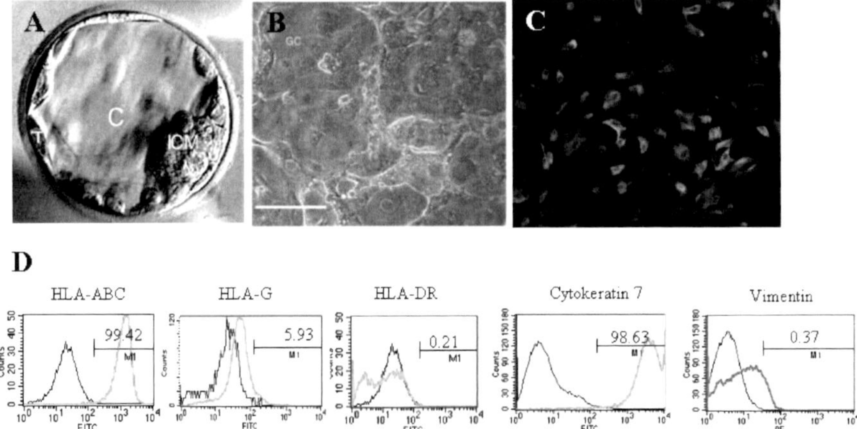

Figure 6. Characterization of trophoblast stem cells. (A) Trophectoderm (T), the inner cell mass (ICM), and blastocystic cavity (C) in the blastocyst. (B) The morphology of cultured trophoblast stem cells. (C) Cytokeratin 7 expression in the cultured trophoblast stem cells using immunofluorescence. (D) The expressions of surface markers for HLA-types, cytokeratin 7 and vimentin in cultured trophoblast stem cells using FACS analysis.

Conclusion

Trophoblast, which is a dynamic cell, derived from the fetus shows different phenotypes and functions when it progresses through the cascade of differentiation during placenta development. Also, it is tightly regulated by several environmental factors within the time and space during differentiation in order to maintain fetus growth and development. The unique characteristics of trophoblasts compared to the other somatic cells are cell-to-cell fusion and invasion even under normal conditions. It originates from fetus but can escape from the immune response of the mother because of its capability to express HLA-class I (e.g. HLA-G) but not HLA-class II. Therefore, these abilities could be studied to further elucidate its mechanism in deciding the cell fate as well as the implantation process. Trophoblast stem cells could be useful materials in future clinical therapy. Although studies on trophoblasts are unlikely to contribute to embryogenesis and placental development, there is an immense potential use of these cells as an in vitro tool to analyze the function of trophoblast. The understanding of the characterization and the potentials of trophoblasts may be critical for the cure of various gynecological diseases.

In summary, much basic research lies ahead before application of trophoblasts or trophoblasts stem cells to patients in a rigorous therapeutic manner is realized. However, mankind will surely benefit enormously by conducting research on these cells.

Abbreviations

bFGF: basic fibroblast growth factor
bHLH: basic helix-loop-helix
BMP: bone morphogenic protein
Cdx2: caudal-related homeobox 2
CP-M: carboxypeptidase-M
CTB: cytotrophoblast cells
Cx: connexin
DAP: tunicamycin-responsive gene, a cathepsin D-like gene
DPPIV: Dipeptidyl peptidase IV
EGF: epidermal growth factor
ERK: Extracellular signal-regulated kinase
ES cells: embryonic stem cells
EVT: endovascular extravillous trophoblast
FAK: focal adhesion kinase
FGF: fibroblast growth factor
FLIP: FLICE-like inhibitory protein (FLIP),
GJIC: gap junctional intercellular communication
GTN: gestational trophoblastic neoplasia
hCG: human chorionic gonadotrophin
HGF: hepatocyte growth factor
HIF: hypoxia inducible factor
HO: heme oxygenase

HSPGs: heparan sulfate proteoglycans
ICAM: intercellular adhesion molecule
ICM: inner cell mass
IGF: insulin-like growth factor
IUGR: intrauterine growth restriction
Jak-Stat: Janus kinase-signal transducers and activators of transcription
KIR: killer-immunoglobulin-like receptors
LIF: leukemia inhibitory factor
M-CSF: Macrophage colony-stimulating factor
MAPK: mitogen-activated protein kinase
Mel-CAM: melanoma cell adhesion molecule
MHC: major histocompatibility complex
MMPs: matrix metalloproteinsase
MUC: Mucin
NK: natural killer
PAI: plasminogen activator inhibitor
PBK-1: glucocorticoid-induced kinase,
PCNA: proliferating cell nuclear antigen
PI3K: phosphatidylinositol 3-kinase
PlGF: placental growth factor
PPAR: nuclear hormone receptor peroxisome proliferator activated receptor
ROCK: Rho kinase
RTK-MAPK: receptor-associated tyrosine kinase-mitogen-activated protein kinase
SOCS: suppressor of cytokine signaling
T-DMR: differentially methylated region
TB: trophoblasts
TGF-beta: transforming growth factor beta
TIMPs: plasminogen activators and tissue inhibitors
TLRs: Toll-like receptors
TS cells: trophoblast stem cells
uPA: urokinase-type plasminogen activator
VEGF: vascular endothelial growth factor

References

[1] Moore, KL; Persaud, TVN. The developing human: clinically oriented embryology. 8th ed. Philadelphia, Saunders Elsevier, 2008.

[2] Horne, AW; White, JO; Lalani, EN. The endometrium and embryo implantation. A receptive endometrium depends on more than hormonal influences. *BMJ.*, 2000, 321(7272), 1301-1302.

[3] Benirschke, K; Kaufmann, P. *Pathology of the Human Placenta*, 4th ed. New York, 2000.

[4] Fazleabas, AT; Kim, JJ; Strakova, Z. Implantation: embryonic signals and the modulation of the uterine environment--a review. *Placenta*, 2004, 25 Suppl A, S26-31.

[5] Köbel, M; Pohl, G; Schmitt, WD; Hauptmann, S; Wang, TL; Shih, IeM. Activation of mitogen-activated protein kinase is required for migration and invasion of placental site trophoblastic tumor. *Am J Pathol.*, 2005, 167(3), 879-885.

[6] Burleigh, AR. Of germ cells, trophoblasts, and cancer stem cells. *Integr Cancer Ther.*, 2008, 7(4), 276-281.

[7] Minas, V; Loutradis, D; Makrigiannakis, A. Factors controlling blastocyst implantation. *Reprod Biomed Online*, 2005, 10(2), 205-216.

[8] Blomberg, L; Hashizume, K; Viebahn, C. Blastocyst elongation, trophoblastic differentiation, and embryonic pattern formation. *Reproduction*, 2008, 135(2), 181-195. Review.

[9] Knöfler, M; Simmons, DG; Lash, GE; Harris, LK; Armant, DR. Regulation of trophoblast invasion - a workshop report. *Placenta*, 2008, 29 Suppl A, S26-28.

[10] Gude, NM; Roberts, CT; Kalionis, B; King, RG. Growth and function of the normalhuman placenta. *Thromb Res.*, 2004, 114(5-6), 397-407. Review.

[11] Douglas, GC; Vandevoort, C; Kumar, P; Chang, TC; Golos, TG. Trophoblast Stem Cells:Models for Investigating Trophectoderm Differentiation and Placental Development. *Endocr Rev.*, 2009 Mar 18. [Epub ahead of print]

[12] Rossant, J. Stem cells and lineage development in the mammalian blastocyst. *Reprod Fertil Dev.*, 2007, 19(1), 111-118. Review.

[13] Oda, M; Shiota, K; Tanaka, S. Trophoblast stem cells. *Methods Enzymol.*, 2006, 419, 387-400. Review.

[14] Schumacher, A; Brachwitz, N; Sohr, S; Engeland, K; Langwisch, S; Dolaptchieva, M; Alexander, T; Taran, A; Malfertheiner, SF; Costa, SD; Zimmermann, G; Nitschke, C; Volk, HD; Alexander, H; Gunzer, M; Zenclussen, AC. Human chorionic gonadotropin attracts regulatory T cells into the fetal-maternal interface during early human pregnancy. *J Immunol.*, 2009, 182(9), 5488-5497.

[15] Fishel, SB; Edwards, RG; Evans, CJ. Human chorionic gonadotropin secreted by preimplantation embryos cultured in vitro. *Science*, 1984, 223(4638), 816-818.

[16] Winterhager, E; Kaufmann, P; Gruemmer, R. Cell-cell-communication during placental development and possible implications for trophoblast proliferation and differentiation. *Placenta*, 2000, 21 Suppl A, S61-S68.

[17] Guzeloglu-Kayisli, O; Kayisli, UA; Taylor, HS. The role of growth factors and cytokines during implantation: endocrine and paracrine interactions. *Semin Reprod Med.*, 2009, 27(1), 62-79.

[18] Imudia, AN; Kilburn, BA; Petkova, A; Edwin, SS; Romero, R; Armant, DR. Expression of heparin-binding EGF-like growth factor in term chorionic villous explants and its role in trophoblast survival. *Placenta*, 2008, 29(9), 784-789.

[19] Tapia, A; Salamonsen, LA; Manuelpillai, U; Dimitriadis, E. Leukemia inhibitory factor promotes human first trimester extravillous trophoblast adhesion to extracellular matrix and secretion of tissue inhibitor of metalloproteinases-1 and -2. *Hum Reprod.*, 2008, 23(8), 1724-1732.

[20] Takahashi, Y; Takahashi, M; Carpino, N; Jou, ST; Chao, JR; Tanaka, S; Shigeyoshi, Y; Parganas, E; Ihle, JN. Leukemia inhibitory factor regulates trophoblast giant cell differentiation via Janus kinase 1-signal transducer and activator of transcription 3-suppressor of cytokine signaling 3 pathway. *Mol Endocrinol.*, 2008, 22(7), 1673-1681.

[21] Lunghi, L; Ferretti, ME; Medici, S; Biondi, C; Vesce, F. Control of human trophoblast function. *Reprod Biol Endocrinol.*, 2007, 5, 6-19. Review.

[22] Das, C; Kumar, VS; Gupta, S; Kumar, S. Network of cytokines, integrins and hormones in human trophoblast cells. *J Reprod Immunol.*, 2002, 53(1-2), 257-268.

[23] Fitzgerald, JS; Busch, S; Wengenmayer, T; Foerster, K; de la Motte, T; Poehlmann, TG; Markert, UR. Signal transduction in trophoblast invasion. *Chem Immunol Allergy*, 2005, 88, 181-199. Review.

[24] Hiden, U; Bilban, M; Knöfler, M; Desoye, G. Kisspeptins and the placenta:regulation of trophoblast invasion. *Rev Endocr Metab Disord.*, 2007, 8(1), 31-39. Review.

[25] Makri, A; Pissimissis, N; Lembessis, P; Polychronakos, C; Koutsilieris, M. The kisspeptin (KiSS-1)/GPR54 system in cancer biology. *Cancer Treat Rev.*, 2008, 34(8), 682-92.

[26] Huppertz, B; Frank, HG; Kingdom, JC; Reister, F; Kaufmann, P. Villous cytotrophoblast regulation of the syncytial apoptotic cascade in the human placenta. *Histochem Cell Biol.*, 1998, 110(5), 495-508.

[27] James, JL; Stone, PR; Chamley, LW. Cytotrophoblast differentiation in the first trimester of pregnancy: evidence for separate progenitors of extravillous trophoblasts and syncytiotrophoblast. *Reproduction.*, 2005, 130(1), 95-103.

[28] Aschkenazi, S; Straszewski, S; Verwer, KM; Foellmer, H; Rutherford, T; Mor, G. Differential regulation and function of the Fas/Fas ligand system in human trophoblast cells. *Biol Reprod.*, 2002, 66(6), 1853-1861.

[29] Hsu, WL; Chen, YH; Chao, KC; Chang, SP; Tsui, KH; Li, HY; Sung, YJ. Anti-fas activating antibody enhances trophoblast outgrowth on endometrial epithelial cells by induction of P38 MAPK/JNK-mediated apoptosis. *Placenta*, 2008, 29(4), 338-46.

[30] Armant, DR. Blastocysts don't go it alone. Extrinsic signals fine-tune the intrinsic developmental program of trophoblast cells. *Dev Biol.*, 2005, 280(2), 260-280.

[31] Roberts, RM; Ezashi, T; Das, P. Trophoblast gene expression: transcription factors in the specification of early trophoblast. *Reprod Biol Endocrinol.*, 2004, 2, 47-55. Review.

[32] Hattori, N; Nishino, K; Ko, YG; Hattori, N; Ohgane, J; Tanaka, S; Shiota, K. Epigenetic control of mouse Oct-4 gene expression in embryonic stem cells and trophoblast stem cells. *J Biol Chem.*, 2004, 279(17), 17063-17069.

[33] Janatpour, MJ; McMaster, MT; Genbacev, O; Zhou, Y; Dong, J; Cross, JC; Israel, MA; Fisher, SJ. Id-2 regulates critical aspects of human cytotrophoblast differentiation, invasion and migration. *Development*, 2000, 127(3), 549-558.

[34] Cross, JC; Baczyk, D; Dobric, N; Hemberger, M; Hughes, M; Simmons, DG; Yamamoto, H; Kingdom, JC. Genes, development and evolution of the placenta. *Placenta*, 2003, 24(2-3), 123-130. Review.

[35] Aplin, JD; Jones, CJ; Harris, LK. Adhesion molecules in human trophoblast – a review. I. Villous trophoblast. *Placenta*, 2009, 30(4), 293-298.

[36] Pollheimer, J; Knöfler, M. Signalling pathways regulating the invasive differentiation of human trophoblasts: a review. *Placenta*, 2005, 26 Suppl A, S21-30. Review.

[37] Morrish, DW; Dakour, J; Li, H. Life and death in the placenta: new peptides and genes regulating human syncytiotrophoblast and extravillous cytotrophoblast lineage formation and renewal. *Curr Protein Pept Sci.*, 2001, 2(3), 245-259. Review.

[38] Smith, AN; Carter, QL; Kniss, DA; Brown, TL. Characterization of a TGFbeta-responsive human trophoblast-derived cell line. *Placenta*, 2001, 22(5), 425-431.

[39] Morrish, DW; Dakour, J; Li, H. Functional regulation of human trophoblast differentiation. *J Reprod Immunol.*, 1998, 39(1-2), 179-195. Review.

[40] Cohen, M; Bischof, P. Factors regulating trophoblast invasion. *Gynecol Obstet Invest.*, 2007, 64(3), 126-130.

[41] Zhao, MR; Qiu, W; Li, YX; Zhang, ZB; Li, D; Wang, YL. Dual effect of transforming growth factor beta1 on cell adhesion and invasion in human placenta trophoblast cells. *Reproduction*, 2006, 132(2), 333-341.

[42] Caniggia, I; Mostachfi, H; Winter, J; Gassmann, M; Lye, SJ; Kuliszewski, M; Post, M. Hypoxia-inducible factor-1 mediates the biological effects of oxygen on human trophoblast differentiation through TGFbeta(3). *J Clin Invest.*, 2000, 105(5), 577-587.

[43] Red-Horse, K; Drake, PM; Fisher, SJ. Human pregnancy: the role of chemokine networks at the fetal-maternal interface. *Expert Rev Mol Med.*, 2004, 6(11), 1-14. Review.

[44] Malassiné, A; Cronier, L. Involvement of gap junctions in placental functions and development. *Biochim Biophys Acta.*, 2005, 1719(1-2), 117-124.

[45] Craven, CM; Morgan, T; Ward, K. Decidual spiral artery remodelling begins before cellular interaction with cytotrophoblasts. *Placenta*, 1998, 19(4), 241-252.

[46] Lyall, F. Priming and remodelling of human placental bed spiral arteries during pregnancy--a review. *Placenta*, 2005, 26 Suppl A, S31-36. Review.

[47] Lyall, F; Simpson, H; Bulmer, JN; Barber, A; Robson, SC. Transforming growth factor-beta expression in human placenta and placental bed in third trimester normal pregnancy, preeclampsia, and fetal growth restriction. *Am J Pathol.*, 2001, 159(5), 1827-1838.

[48] Chaddha, V; Viero, S; Huppertz, B; Kingdom, J. Developmental biology of the placenta and the origins of placental insufficiency. *Semin Fetal Neonatal Med.*, 2004, 9(5), 357-369. Review.

[49] Irminger-Finger, I; Jastrow, N; Irion, O. Preeclampsia: a danger growing in disguise. *Int J Biochem Cell Biol.*, 2008, 40(10), 1979-1983.

[50] Regnault, TR; de Vrijer, B; Galan, HL; Davidsen, ML; Trembler, KA; Battaglia, FC; Wilkening, RB; Anthony, RV. The relationship between transplacental O2 diffusion and placental expression of PlGF, VEGF and their receptors in a placental insufficiency model of fetal growth restriction. *J Physiol.*, 2003, 550(Pt 2), 641-656.

[51] Dai, J; Rabie, AB. VEGF: an essential mediator of both angiogenesis and endochondral ossification. *J Dent Res.*, 2007, 86(10), 937-950. Review.

[52] Abbott, BD; Buckalew, AR. Placental defects in ARNT-knockout conceptus correlate with localized decreases in VEGF-R2, Ang-1, and Tie-2. *Dev Dyn.*, 2000, 219(4), 526-538.

[53] Cowden Dahl, KD; Fryer, BH; Mack, FA; Compernolle, V; Maltepe, E; Adelman, DM; Carmeliet, P; Simon, MC. Hypoxia-inducible factors 1alpha and 2alpha regulate trophoblast differentiation. *Mol Cell Biol.*, 2005, 25(23), 10479-10491.

[54] Ietta, F; Wu, Y; Winter, J; Xu, J; Wang, J; Post, M; Caniggia, I. Dynamic HIF1A regulation during human placental development. *Biol Reprod.*, 2006, 75(1), 112-121.

[55] Li, H; Gu, B; Zhang, Y; Lewis, DF; Wang, Y. Hypoxia-induced increase in soluble Flt-1 production correlates with enhanced oxidative stress in trophoblast cells from the human placenta. *Placenta*, 2005, 26(2-3), 210-217.

[56] Ahmad, S; Ahmed, A. Elevated placental soluble vascular endothelial growth factor receptor-1 inhibits angiogenesis in preeclampsia. *Circ Res.*, 2004, 95(9), 884-891.

[57] Noris, M; Perico, N; Remuzzi, G. Mechanisms of disease: Pre-eclampsia. *Nat Clin Pract Nephrol.*, 2005, 1(2), 98-114.

[58] Kingdom, JC; Kaufmann, P. Oxygen and placental vascular development. *Adv Exp Med Biol.*, 1999, 474, 259-275. Review.

[59] Munaut, C; Lorquet, S; Pequeux, C; Blacher, S; Berndt, S; Frankenne, F; Foidart, JM. Hypoxia is responsible for soluble vascular endothelial growth factor receptor-1 (VEGFR-1) but not for soluble endoglin induction in villous trophoblast. *Hum Reprod.*, 2008, 23(6), 1407-1415.

[60] Regnault, TR; Galan, HL; Parker, TA; Anthony, RV. Placental development in normal and compromised pregnancies-- a review. *Placenta*, 2002, 23 Suppl A, S119-S129.

[61] Lockwood, CJ; Toti, P; Arcuri, F; Norwitz, E; Funai, EF; Huang, ST; Buchwalder, LF; Krikun, G; Schatz, F. Thrombin regulates soluble fms-like tyrosine kinase-1 (sFlt-1) expression in first trimester decidua: implications for preeclampsia. Am *J Pathol.*, 2007, 170(4), 1398-1405.

[62] Goldman-Wohl, D; Yagel, S. Regulation of trophoblast invasion: from normal implantation to pre-eclampsia. *Mol Cell Endocrinol.*, 2002, 187(1-2), 233-238. Review.

[63] Rampersad, R; Nelson, DM. Trophoblast biology, responses to hypoxia and placental dysfunction in preeclampsia. *Front Biosci.*, 2007, 12, 2447-2456.Review.

[64] Kaufmann, P; Black, S; Huppertz, B. Endovascular trophoblast invasion: implications for the pathogenesis of intrauterine growth retardation and preeclampsia. *Biol Reprod.*, 2003, 69(1), 1-7.

[65] Harris, LK; Jones, CJ; Aplin, JD. Adhesion Molecules in Human Trophoblast – A Review. II. Extravillous Trophoblast. *Placenta*, 2009, 30(4), 299-304.

[66] Bauer, S; Pollheimer, J; Hartmann, J; Husslein, P; Aplin, JD; Knöfler, M. Tumor necrosis factor-alpha inhibits trophoblast migration through elevation of plasminogen activator inhibitor-1 in first-trimester villous explant cultures. *J Clin Endocrinol Metab.*, 2004, 89(2), 812-822.

[67] Shyu, MK; Lin, MC; Liu, CH; Fu, YR; Shih, JC; Lee, CN; Chen, HY; Huang, J; Huang, MC; Hsieh, FJ. MUC1 expression is increased during human placental development and suppresses trophoblast-like cell invasion in vitro. *Biol Reprod.*, 2008, 79(2), 233-239.

[68] Merviel, P; Challier, JC; Carbillon, L; Foidart, JM; Uzan, S. The role of integrins in human embryo implantation. *Fetal Diagn Ther.*, 2001, 16(6), 364-371.

[69] Zhou, Y; Damsky, CH; Chiu, K; Roberts, JM; Fisher, SJ. Preeclampsia is associated with abnormal expression of adhesion molecules by invasive cytotrophoblasts. *J Clin Invest.*, 1993, 91(3), 950-960.

[70] Iwaki, T; Yamamoto, K; Matsuura, T; Sugimura, M; Kobayashi, T; Kanayama, N. Alteration of integrins under hypoxic stress in early placenta and choriocarcinoma cell line BeWo. *Gynecol Obstet Invest.*, 2004, 57(4), 196-203.

[71] Chakraborty, C; Gleeson, LM; McKinnon, T; Lala, PK. Regulation of human trophoblast migration and invasiveness. *Can J Physiol Pharmacol.*, 2002, 80(2), 116-124. Review.

[72] Abe, E; Matsubara, K; Oka, K; Kusanagi, Y; Ito, M. Cytokine regulation of intercellular adhesion molecule-1 expression on trophoblasts in preeclampsia. *Gynecol Obstet Invest.*, 2008, 66(1), 27-33.

[73] Bischof, P. Endocrine, paracrine and autocrine regulation of trophoblastic metalloproteinases. *Early Pregnancy*, 2001, 5(1), 30-31.

[74] Fujiwara, H; Higuchi, T; Sato, Y; Nishioka, Y; Zeng, BX; Yoshioka, S; Tatsumi, K; Ueda, M; Maeda, M. Regulation of human extravillous trophoblast function by membrane-bound peptidases. *Biochim Biophys Acta.*, 2005, 1751(1), 26-32.

[75] Fujiwara, H. Membrane-bound peptidases regulate human extravillous trophoblast invasion. *Placenta*, 2007, 28 Suppl A, S70-75.

[76] Nishioka, Y; Higuchi, T; Sato, Y; Yoshioka, S; Tatsumi, K; Fujiwara, H; Fujii, S. Human migrating extravillous trophoblasts express a cell surface peptidase, carboxypeptidase-M. *Mol Hum Reprod.*, 2003, 9(12), 799-806.

[77] Jarvenpaa, J; Vuoristo, JT; Savolainen, ER; Ukkola, O; Vaskivuo, T; Ryynanen, M. Altered expression of angiogenesis-related placental genes in pre-eclampsia associated with intrauterine growth restriction. *Gynecol Endocrinol.*, 2007, 23(6), 351-355.

[78] Bilban, M; Haslinger, P; Prast, J; Klinglmüller, F; Woelfel, T; Haider, S; Sachs, A; Otterbein, LE; Desoye, G; Hiden, U; Wagner, O; Knöfler, M. Identification of novel trophoblast invasion-related genes: heme oxygenase-1 controls motility via peroxisome proliferator-activated receptor gamma. *Endocrinology*, 2009, 150(2), 1000-1013.

[79] Bilban, M; Head, S; Desoye, G; Quaranta, V. DNA microarrays: a novel approach to investigate genomics in trophoblast invasion--a review. *Placenta*, 2000, 21 Suppl A, S99-105. Review.

[80] Fournier, T; Handschuh, K; Tsatsaris, V; Guibourdenche, J; Evain-Brion, D. Role of nuclear receptors and their ligands in human trophoblast invasion. *J Reprod Immunol.*, 2008, 77(2), 161-170.

[81] Yeshaya, J; Amir, I; Rimon, A; Freedman, J; Shohat, M; Avivi, L. Microdeletion syndromes disclose replication timing alterations of genes unrelated to the missing DNA. *Mol Cytogenet.*, 2009, 2, 11-22.

[82] Naruse, K; Lash, GE; Innes, BA; Otun, HA; Searle, RF; Robson, SC; Bulmer, JN. Localization of matrix metalloproteinase (MMP)-2, MMP-9 and tissue inhibitors for MMPs (TIMPs) in uterine natural killer cells in early human pregnancy. *Hum Reprod.*, 2009, 24(3), 553-561.

[83] Hu, Y; Dutz, JP; MacCalman, CD; Yong, P; Tan, R; von Dadelszen, P. Decidual NK cells alter in vitro first trimester extravillous cytotrophoblast migration: a role for IFN-gamma. *J Immunol.*, 2006, 177(12), 8522-8530.

[84] Koga, K; Aldo, PB; Mor, G. Toll-like receptors and pregnancy: Trophoblast as modulators of the immune response. *J Obstet Gynaecol Res.*, 2009, 35(2), 191-202.

[85] Mor, G. Inflammation and pregnancy: the role of toll-like receptors in trophoblast-immune interaction. *Ann N Y Acad Sci.*, 2008, 1127, 121-128. Review

[86] Hanna, J; Goldman-Wohl, D; Hamani, Y; Avraham, I; Greenfield, C; Natanson-Yaron, S; Prus, D; Cohen-Daniel, L; Arnon, TI; Manaster, I; Gazit, R; Yutkin, V; Benharroch, D; Porgador, A; Keshet, E; Yagel, S; Mandelboim, O. Decidual NK cells regulate key developmental processes at the human fetal-maternal interface. *Nat Med.*, 2006, 12(9), 1065-1074.

[87] Goldman-Wohl, D; Yagel, S. NK cells and pre-eclampsia. *Reprod Biomed Online.*, 2008, 16(2), 227-31. Review

[88] Rizzo, R; Melchiorri, L; Stignani, M; Baricordi, OR. HLA-G expression is a fundamental prerequisite to pregnancy. *Hum Immunol.*, 2007, 68(4), 244-250.

[89] van der Meer, A; Lukassen, HG; van Cranenbroek, B; Weiss, EH; Braat, DD; van Lierop, MJ; Joosten, I. Soluble HLA-G promotes Th1-type cytokine production by cytokine-activated uterine and peripheral natural killer cells. *Mol Hum Reprod.*, 2007, 13(2), 123-133.

[90] Cole, LA; Khanlian, SA. Hyperglycosylated hCG: a variant with separate biological functions to regular hCG. *Mol Cell Endocrinol.*, 2007, 260-262, 228-236.

[91] Poehlmann, TG; Fitzgerald, JS; Meissner, A; Wengenmayer, T; Schleussner, E; Friedrich, K; Markert, UR. Trophoblast invasion: tuning through LIF, signalling via Stat3. *Placenta*, 2005, 26 Suppl A, S37-41.

[92] Thomson, JA; Kalishman, J; Golos, TG; Durning, M; Harris, CP; Becker, RA; Hearn, JP. Isolation of a primate embryonic stem cell line. *Proc Natl Acad Sci*, U S A., 1995, 92(17), 7844-7848.

[93] Adjaye, J; Huntriss, J; Herwig, R; BenKahla, A; Brink, TC; Wierling, C; Hultschig, C; Groth, D; Yaspo, ML; Picton, HM; Gosden, RG; Lehrach, H. Primary differentiation in the human blastocyst: comparative molecular portraits of inner cell mass and trophectoderm cells. *Stem Cells.*, 2005, 23(10), 1514-1525.

[94] Wen, F; Tynan, JA; Cecena, G; Williams, R; Múnera, J; Mavrothalassitis, G; Oshima, RG. Ets2 is required for trophoblast stem cell self-renewal. *Dev Biol.*, 2007, 312(1), 284-299.

[95] Hattori, N; Imao, Y; Nishino, K; Hattori, N; Ohgane, J; Yagi, S; Tanaka, S; Shiota, K. Epigenetic regulation of Nanog gene in embryonic stem and trophoblast stem cells. *Genes Cells*, 2007, 12(3), 387-396.

[96] Babaie, Y; Herwig, R; Greber, B; Brink, TC; Wruck, W; Groth, D; Lehrach, H; Burdon, T; Adjaye, J. Analysis of Oct4-dependent transcriptional networks regulating self-renewal and pluripotency in human embryonic stem cells. *Stem Cells*, 2007, 25(2), 500-510.

[97] Niwa, H; Toyooka, Y; Shimosato, D; Strumpf, D; Takahashi, K; Yagi, R; Rossant, J. Interaction between Oct3/4 and Cdx2 determines trophectoderm differentiation.*Cell*, 2005, 123(5), 917-929.

[98] Moore, H; Udayashankar, R; Aflatoonian, B. Stem cells for reproductive medicine. *Mol Cell Endocrinol.*, 2008, 288(1-2), 104-110.

[99] Takahashi, Y; Dominici, M; Swift, J; Nagy, C; Ihle, JN. Trophoblast stem cells rescue placental defect in SOCS3-deficient mice. *J Biol Chem.*, 2006, 281(17), 11444-11445.

[100] Harun, R; Ruban, L; Matin, M; Draper, J; Jenkins, NM; Liew, GC; Andrews, PW; Li, TC; Laird, SM; Moore, HD. Cytotrophoblast stem cell lines derived from human embryonic stem cells and their capacity to mimic invasive implantation events. *Hum Reprod.*, 2006, 21(6), 1349-1358.

In: Human Placenta: Structure and Development... ISBN: 978-1-60876-457-0
Editors: E. Berven, et al. pp. 79-123 © 2010 Nova Science Publishers, Inc.

Chapter III

Placental Insulin-Like Growth and Regulatory Factors and Their Roles in Human Prenatal Growth and Development

Mrinal K. Sanyal, Shai Pri-Paz and Ronald J. Wapner
Department of Obstetrics and Gynecology, Columbia University Medical Center, 622W, 168th Street, New York, NY.

Abstract

The placenta plays a major role in regulating fetal growth and development during human pregnancy. The placental development correlates with the fetal growth. Insulin like growth factors (IGF-1 and -2) are essential growth factors promoting cellular multiplication for growth and differentiation of the placental and fetal tissues. Placenta is a major source of IGFs during pregnancy. In addition, IGF-binding proteins (BP -1, -3 and -4) and metalloproteinase enzymes (pregnancy associated plasma protein A; PAPP-A and A Disintegrin and Metalloproteinase 12s; ADAM-12s) are abundantly produced and are quantifiable in maternal sera during pregnancy. The levels of these factors in maternal sera vary with the progression of normal pregnancy, and may be reduced in various adverse pregnancy conditions. It is suggested that the placenta contributes to IGF production and its biosynthesis is regulated by the "IGF-axis" involving growth hormone releasing factor ghrelin (GHRL) and a structurally variant growth hormone (GH-2) during pregnancy. Unlike production of IGFs during the postnatal period which is an endocrine process with the participation of the hypothalamus, pituitary and liver, generation of IGFs during the prenatal periods to a large extent is by paracrine-autocrine processes. The placenta and fetal membranes produce IGF-binding proteins (IGF-BPs) and metalloproteinases (PAPP-A and ADAM-12s) and active and free IGFs are generated by proteolytic separation of IGFs and BPs. Availability of free IGFs which may bind with its cellular receptors for multiplication and differentiation of cells is required for prenatal development. PAPP-A is released in plasma as a complex of proform of eosinophil major basic protein (pro-MBP). The proteolytic activity of PAPP-A is presumably regulated by binding with pro-MBP which inhibits its proteinase activity. A variety of genes associated with these factors are expressed in placental and other conceptus tissues and their relative expression (mRNA and proteins) may be related to adverse pregnancy outcomes. In addition, single nucleotide polymorphisms (SNPs) and mutations which are variations of nucleotide sequences of genes may affect the functions of cells and differentiation and development of the fetus and placenta. Thus, both biosynthesis and bioavailability of IGFs may play a critical role in normal and abnormal placental and fetal development during pregnancy, and associated with the adverse outcomes, including intrauterine fetal growth retardation (IUGR) and premature births which significantly influence neonatal survival and morbidity, and subsequent postnatal life.

1. Introduction

The human placenta plays a significant role in fetal development during pregnancy. Among many functions of the placenta, generation of diverse growth factors and their regulation and transport into the fetal compartment are now recognized to be an important placental function. Among the growth factors, insulin like growth factors -1 and -2 (IGF1 and IGF2), play critical roles in the development, differentiation and growth (increase in cell number, size and weight) of the placenta and fetus. The IGF1 specifically promotes growth and differentiation of fetal primordial cells and tissues into organs (e. g., muscle, bone and neural tissues) and IGF2 influences placental differentiation and functions. Placental production of such growth and regulatory factors is important from an early gestation period until the fetal organs are differentiated and functionally competent. In this chapter, the generation of IGFs and their regulation (biosynthesis and bioavailability) during pregnancy, and how these processes may be related to the adverse pregnancy outcomes will be discussed.

2. Progressive Development of the Placenta and Embryo-Fetus

(a) Embryo Implantation and Placental Differentiation

The human embryo at the blastocyst stage (approximately 200 cells) implants within the maternal uterine tissues by 7 days post coitus (1-3). The embryoblast (inner cell mass) of the blastocyst stage embryo develops into fetus, umbilical cord and amnion of the conceptus and the outer trophectoderm cells differentiate into placenta and fetal membranes. The trophectoderm cells develop into chorionic villi with a continuous layer of proliferative cytotrophoblast cells (Langhans) which becomes a multinucleated cellular layer (syncytiotrophoblast). The syncytiotrophoblast is the interface between the fetal and maternal compartments and it has no regenerative potential. The chorionic villi develop fetal circulation by the 5th week and are responsible for fetal nutritional and oxygen exchanges during pregnancy. The primordial cytotrophoblast cells also differentiate into another population of migratory and invasive cells, extravillous trophoblast cells with no syncytial fusion.

The implanting embryo is subdivided anatomically into two poles: implantation (basal chorion) and anti-implantation (capsular chorion) poles (2-3). Primordial chorionic villi cells initially surround both the anti-implantation (chorion frondosum; CF) and implantation (capsular chorionic frondosum) poles (Figure 1; Left). Approximately by the 3rd week post conception, cells and tissues at the anti-implantation pole begin to focally dislodge and spreads laterally covering nearly 70% of the CF with the progress of pregnancy. The trophoblast cells of the CF at the anti-implantation pole, decidual cells lining the uterine cavity (UC), migratory extravillous trophoblast cells, maternal white blood cells, and fetal erythroblasts may populate the uterine cavity at this period (Figure 1; Right).

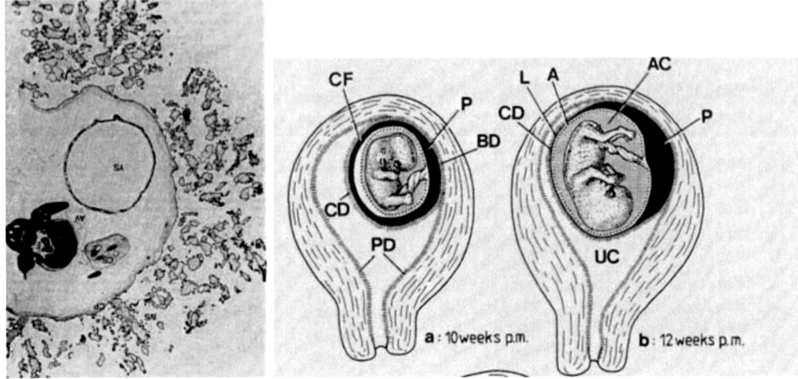

Figure 1. Placental development and differentiation during the first trimester of pregnancy. *Left*: Section of embryo-placenta at 4th wk gestation with extended branching primordial villi. The villi cells at the anti-implantation pole are shed with the progress in fetal-placental development. *Right*: By the 10th & 12th wk of gestation, cells of the chorionic frondosum (CF) over capsular decidua (CD) at the anti-implantation pole are dislodged focally, and those at the implantation pole form the placenta (P) apposed to basal decidua (BD). The uterine cavity is lined by parietal decidual (PD) cells. (Benrischke, et al., 2-3)

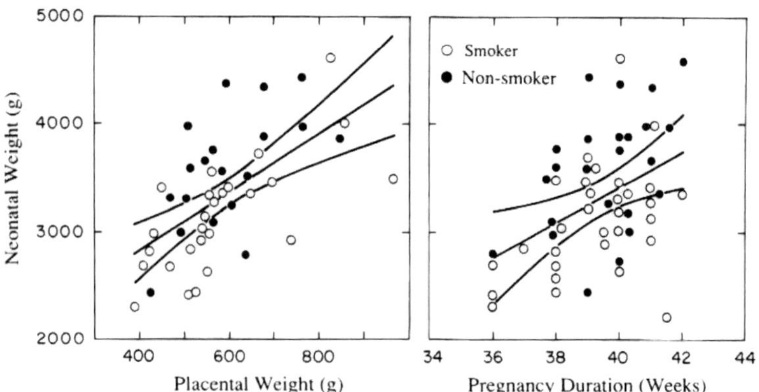

Figure 2. Scatter diagrams of birth weights of neonates and placentas of smoker and non-smoker mothers. *Left*: The regression lines (and 95% confidence intervals) of the neonatal birth weights significantly correlated with placental weight. *Right:* Birth weight of neonate and placenta were also correlated to pregnancy duration and smoke exposure (4).

The fetus by 10-12 weeks of pregnancy is within the fluid-filled amniotic cavity (AC) lined by amnion (A) and chorion leave (L) cells. The extravillous trophoblast cells originate from the chorionic villi. They are proliferative, migratory and invasive, and are found in the chorionic plate, basal plate, and among decidual tissues. They may also populate the utero-placental arterial outlets and enter the arterial lumen by a side route and migrate against the blood flow adhering to the endothelium of the arterial walls. These cells do not invade into venous outlets. Aggregation of such trophoblast cells in the spiral arteries is associated with loss of elasticity of smooth muscle cells of the arterial wall making it rigid and wider as much as 2000 μm in diameter during pregnancy (2). This is associated with the loss of elasticity which is more prominent at the decidual part of the basal plate. Absence of arterial impendence and constriction capability allows a continued delivery of oxygen and nutrients into placental-fetal complex. Aberrations in this process may also contribute to development of preeclampsia- a hypertensive disease of pregnancy.

(b) Relationship of Neonatal and Placental Growth at Delivery and Pregnancy Duration

The conceptus progressively differentiates and grows in size and weight during pregnancy at variable rates determined by multiple factors, including maternal nutrition, pathology of the placenta and availability of growth, regulatory and endocrine factors. The weights of the neonate at birth usually directly correlate with the weight of placenta (Figure 2; left) and with the duration of pregnancy (Figure 2; right) indicating the importance of placental development for fetal growth during pregnancy (4-5). Such a direct correlation of placental and fetal growth is also demonstrated in cases of deleterious maternal cigarette smoke exposure. The deleterious effects of maternal cigarette smoke exposure on fetus-placenta were, in general, dose related. However, reduction in fetal and placental growth was variable by exposure to such toxicity (Figure 2; 4).

(c) Progressive Placental and Fetal Growth and Differentiation during Pregnancy

With the advent of a more precise ultrasound imaging capabilities, monitoring of the progressive human fetal and placental development *in vivo* during the 1st, 2nd and 3rd trimesters of gestation is possible (6-8). Using transabdominal and transvaginal ultrasonographic methods, the progressive development of the placental and fetal organs, and identification of fetal structural anomalies can be made *in utero* non-invasively antenatally (9-12). These methods also allow estimation of the fetal size and weights and measuring biometric anatomical parameters (13-16), generation of 2-D and 3-D images of fetal organs (17- 20) and placental features (21-23) during *in utero* development. These images of fetal and placental tissues permit analysis of their progressive development. In addition, pulse Doppler analysis of blood flow permits assessment of functional competence of the blood vascular system and identification of adverse pregnancies due to abnormalities of blood flow (24-27).

At present, progressive fetal and placental development for each pregnancy can be followed individually by applying such ultrasonographic imaging methods. Biometric data on fetal anatomical parameters (crown rump length, CRL; head circumference, HC; biparietal diameter, BPD; abdominal circumference, AC and femur length, FL) collected at different periods in gestation can assess the fetal growth velocity and individualized growth (weight and size) compared to the standard for the gestational ages. The estimated fetal weight (EFW) and an altered fetal growth potential compared to that of standard (normal) can be determined by such monitoring of pregnancies. The threshold of less than the 10th percentile of expected fetal weight identifies intrauterine growth restricted fetuses (IUGR). These are usually small for gestational age fetuses at birth (SGA; <2500 g birth weight). Similarly, excessive fetal growth can be estimated by such prenatal ultrasound imaging procedures which will produce a large for gestational age (LGA) neonates.

The progressive fetal development could be assessed by different fetal growth models (28-35). Fetal growth is markedly influenced by diverse factors generated by both placental and fetal tissues and by maternal supply of essential requirements for fetal-placental development. In addition, development of the fetus-placenta may also be affected by inherent genomic mutations and involuntary or involuntary deleterious maternal exposure. The growth models may identify IUGR and other disorders of fetal growth by biometric data during different periods of gestation. Disproportionate organogenesis of the fetus can be assessed by 3-D volumetric analysis of different fetal organs (liver, brain, arms, etc.). Widely used anatomic biometric parameters of the fetus obtained by the ultrasonographic imaging for fetal growth assessment are given below:

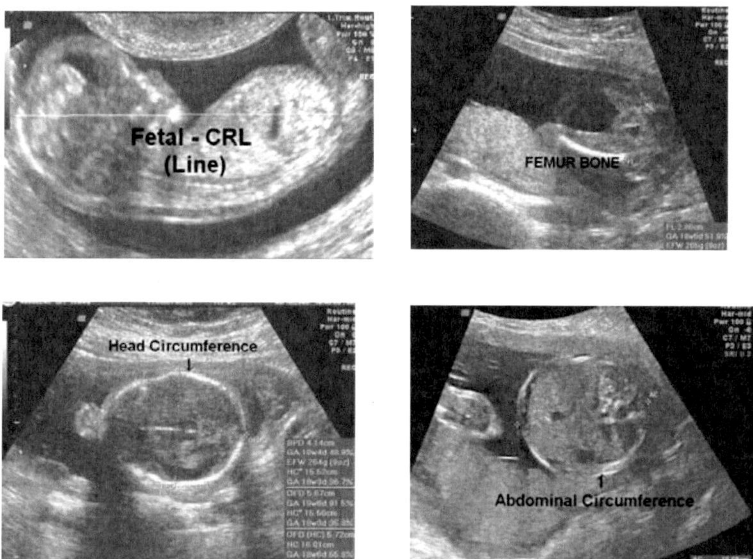

Figure 3. Ultrasonographic images of the developing fetal anatomical biometric parameters. *Upper Panel: Left* – Body length of the fetus during first trimester pregnancy. It is determined by visualizing the fetus sagittally and measuring the crown rump length (CRL; line). *Right*- The femur bone development (FL; white structure); measurement of the shaft without the epiphysis represents femur length. *Lower Panel: Left* - The elliptical outline of the cranium (arrow) is a transverse view of the fetal head. The two cranial measures of fetal growth are calculated, head circumference (HC) and brain biparital diameter (BPD) perpendicular to the fronto-occipital axis. *Right* - Transverse view of the fetal abdomen at the level of liver. Circumference of the abdomen (AC; arrow) and the liver is shown at right angle.

(d) Comparison of Normal and *in utero* Growth Restricted Fetus-Placenta

Multiple factors may induce intrauterine growth restriction (IUGR) and the IUGR process may be symmetric or it may be asymmetric affecting the fetal organs differentially. For example, the fetal head circumference is not initially affected in IUGR cases secondary to placental insufficiency and this phenomenon is known as "brain sparing" effect. Another example of the brain sparing process is observed for maternal exposure to toxic cigarette smoke in which the fetal head circumferences (HC) and femur bone lengths (FL) are apparently not affected. Comparison of slopes of individual biometric parameters: HC, FL, AC, muscle and fat areas of the thigh, estimate of fetal weight and percentage of fat tissue in thigh between groups with exposure and without smoke exposure, revealed that the lean body-mass were significantly affected by smoke (36-38).

The reduced fetal growth in mothers exposed to cigarette smoke selectively affected the AC and peripheral muscle mass with no apparent effect on the HC and FL in fetuses. Selective toxic effects of smoke exposure within the lean body mass and peripheral muscle tissues and a reduced size of the liver resulted in the reduction of the AC. A reduced AC appears to be the most sensitive fetal parameter for growth restriction and dysmorphogenesis. There was a 5-7 fold increase in the lean body mass in cross-sectional area of lean body mass between 19-40 weeks of gestation. However, the increase in the subcutaneous fat mass during the same period was approximately 10-fold greater (36).

Although 2-D analysis of different biometric parameters outlined above may reveal the extent of developmental potential of the conceptus, the 3-D analysis of anatomical parameters and specific organ volumes provide more accurate values for assessing fetal growth disturbances. The structural units of fetal arms and thighs consist of differentiated tissues (e. g., skin, muscle, nerve and bone) derived from the ectoderm and mesoderm (Figure 4; below). These tissues may reflect the deficits of maternal nutrition and the roles of various growth factors (IGF- axis). These fetal tissues are the targets of action for various growth and their regulatory factors promoting growth and differentiation.

Liver and brain volumes assessed by 3-D analysis during the 2nd and 3rd trimesters of pregnancy reveals the differential features of their normal development and that for IUGR (17-20). The 3-D image of the liver volume may predict IUGR. The sensitivity of fetal liver in predicting IUGR was 97.6 % and the specificity 93.9% (17-18). Similarly, 3-D determination of brain and cerebellum volumes (19-20) reveals their *in utero* development characteristics. Sonographic estimates of brain/liver volume ratios have been shown to be a predictor of fetal growth restriction (13). Reduction of liver development in IUGR is more pronounced than the head (brain sparing). Relative reduction of liver and brain volumes are important structural changes during IUGR of the fetus which may be influenced by blood flow to these organs. In addition, the possibility of symmetric and asymmetric reduction in these organs of the fetus induced by different etiologies has been suggested.

Usually, the symmetric IUGRs are related to chromosomal anomalies or infection and the asymmetric conditions are due to placental insufficiencies.

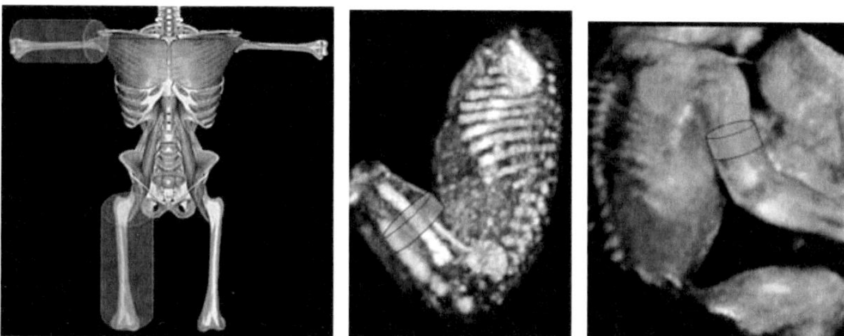

Figure 4. The concept of fractional limb volume analysis is outlined in (left; drawing) showing the limb volume measurement including both bone and soft tissues (arrows). Middle and right figures depict the 3-D reconstructions of the limb units and fetal body for assessment of deviations in *in utero* fetal growth and development (39-41).

Placental features and anomalies

Placental volume is an important parameter reflecting placental function vital to fetal development. The placental volume at the end of first trimester and through the second trimesters of pregnancy has been shown to correlate with growth of the fetus (21-23). Insufficiency in placental functions is associated with reduced distribution of requirements for growth and anomalous development of the fetus. Abnormal placentation, such as, placenta previa and umbilical cord location (insertion) may affect blood supply and fetal development. Placental anomalies of abruption and previa (approximately .5% of pregnancies) are known to be associated with IUGR and other adverse pregnancy conditions. Another placental anomaly of interest is marginal umbilical cord insertion, rather than in the middle of the chorionic plate. An asymmetric placental plate and cord insertion associated with amniotic membrane may also affect the development of the fetus. Thus, ultrasound imaging may now reveal such placental anomalies *in utero* noninvasively while the fetus is developing during pregnancy. Whether these anomalies of placenta may influence fetal development by subnormal placental function (e. g., IGF2 production, nutrition and O_2 transport) affecting normal fetal development is unknown. Some examples of such placental anomalies identified by the sonographic procedures are illustrated below (Figure 5):

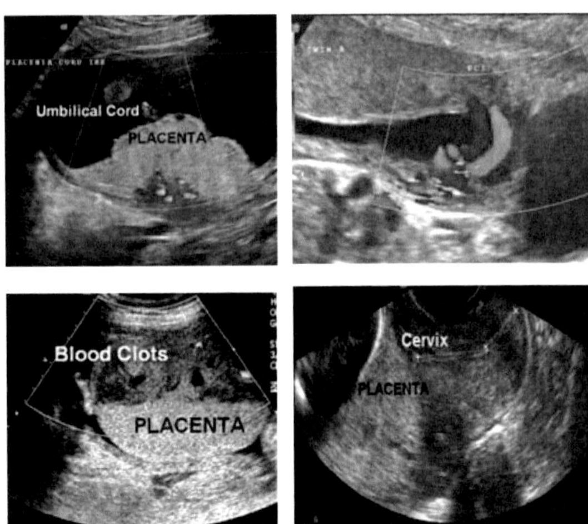

Figure 5. Placenta visualized by ultrasound imaging. *Upper Left:* Normal placenta, image within the view box umbilical cord insertion shown in color. *Upper right*: Anomalous (marginal) cord insertion into placenta in a twin pregnancy. *Lower left*: Abruption (separation) of the placenta from the maternal uterine decidua. A hematoma (blood clots) is associated with placenta may be a cause of premature separation of placenta. *Lower right*: Placenta previa (abnormal placentation) over the cervix covering the internal os. The dotted line marks to cervical canal. (Pri-Paz, S. et al., unpublished).

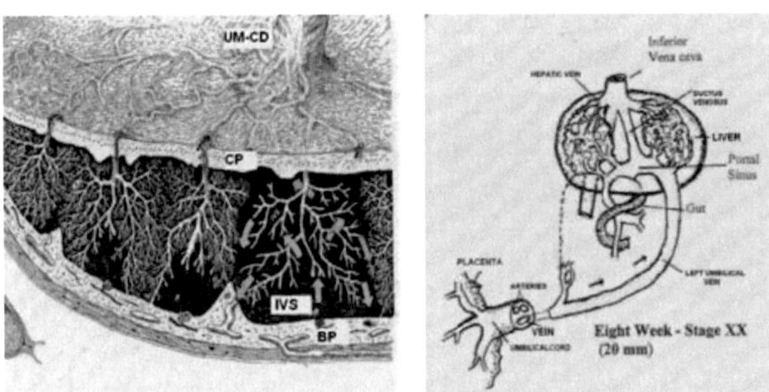

Figure 6. Anatomy of the placental villi and fetal vasculature. *Left*: The diagram shows the umbilical cord (UM-CD) and cross section of the placenta with chorionic plate (CP) facing the fetus and basal plate (BP) attached to the maternal uterine wall. Blood flow in the inter-villous (IVS) space is marked by multiple arrows (2-3). *Right*: Depicts the two arteries of the umbilical cord carrying blood from the fetal heart and one vein from the placenta entering into the fetus (1). The umbilical vein delivers blood rich in various growth factors, nutrients and O_2 from the placenta into the fetus and the two arteries return fetal products into placenta. This vasculature architecture is radically changed at birth in the neonate after separation from the umbilical cord and placenta.

2. Transport of Placental Product into Fetal Compartment

(a) Placental Anatomy and Blood Supply

Human placenta is hemochorial with branching chorionic villi submerged within the inter-villous blood (Figure 6; 1, 3). Diverse products synthesized by cells of the chorionic villi are released into the intervillous spaces (IVS) and also carried by the umbilical vein into the fetal compartment. In addition, blood in the IVS is oxygenated and enriched with substances produced by the maternal system (hormones, antibodies, nutrients). Progressive development of the fetal blood vascular system allows utilization of these products for fetal growth. Well differentiated ductus venosus in the fetus during mid-pregnancy is an important component of fetal vasculature development. It allows preferential distribution of blood to the upper part of the fetus by delivering blood to the left atrium through the foramen ovale. It is a specialized fetal feature for its wellbeing. At present, the biological mechanisms of this regulatory process in the developing fetus remain unclear.

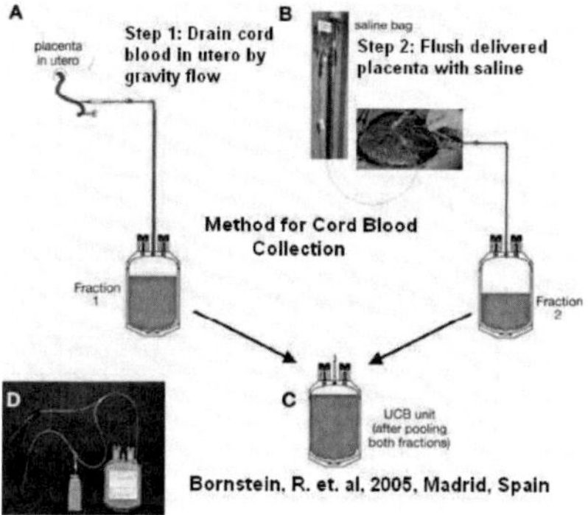

Figure 7. Procedure for umbilical cord blood collection. *Step 1:* The umbilical cord of placenta *in utero* is clamped, transected and cleaned with iodine and alcohol. A 16-gauze needle from the collection bag is inserted into the umbilical vein/artery. Blood is allowed to flow by gravity into a collection bag until the flow is ceased. *Step 2:* The delivered placenta is flushed through large placental vessels with 50 ml of buffered saline (or tissues culture media) and heparin. A large vessel (artery or vein) of the umbilical cord is cannulated for in-flow of saline or culture media hung on a drip stand. A circulatory pump may be incorporated at the out-flow end. This procedure generates cell types (mononuclear and trophoblast) of the umbilical cord. The recovered cells and liquid can be stored frozen (at -80°C or liquid N_2 -156°C).

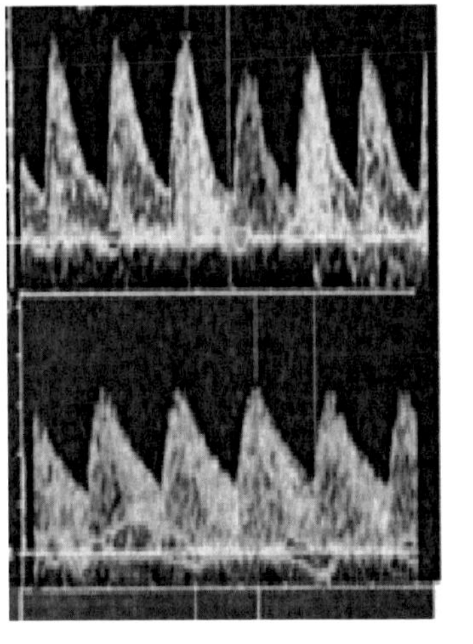

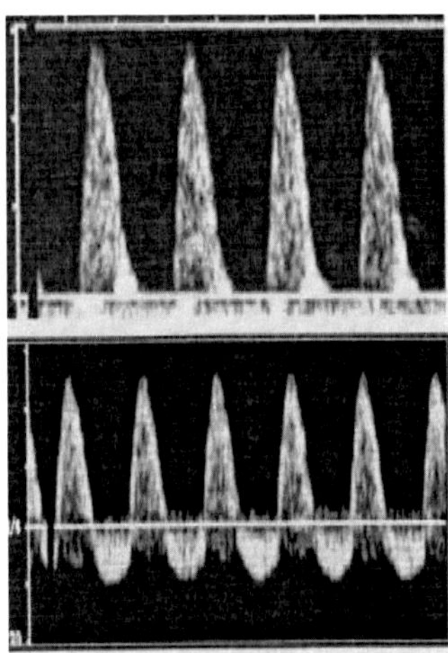

Left Right

Figure 8. Doppler wave form of the umbilical blood vessels during 2nd and 3rd trimester of pregnancy. *Left*: The pattern of relatively high resistance and consistent diastolic blood flow in artery during the 2nd trimester (18 week) (upper panel). Resistance is reduced with the progress of pregnancy and diastolic flow is increased significantly by the 3rd trimester as reflected by a lower systolic/diastolic ratio (lower panel). *Right:* In the pregnancies with severe IUGR due to placental insufficiencies, the Doppler patterns are significantly altered (45-46). The umbilical artery may exhibit an absence of end diastolic (AEDF) blood flow (upper panel) or reversal of end diastolic (REDF) indicating disturbances in fetal circulation due to insufficiencies in placental functions (lower panel).

The placenta often remains within the mother after delivery before expulsion for a short period of time. This period is called the third stage of delivery and may last for about 30 minutes. Blood extracted from the umbilical cord of placenta within the uterus (neonate removed) provides greater yields and also richer in factors. A combination of *in utero* blood collection and a perfusion system for expelled human placenta with buffered saline or tissue culture media using a circulatory pump allows optimal extraction diverse cells and residual umbilical blood as outlined below (42; Figure 7):

The umbilical cord matrix (Wharton's Jelly) and blood are major resources of different types of stem cells. These stem cells may have therapeutic values for some cancers, metabolic diseases and have potential for future therapy for birth defects. Cord blood banks have been established for a long-term preservation of the umbilical cord sera and cells.

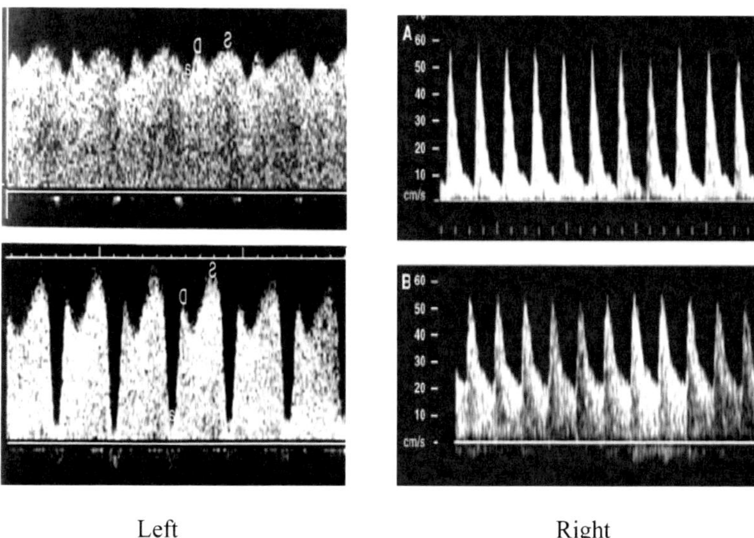

Left Right

Figure 9. (*Left)*: Upper panel depicts the normal flow pattern of the ductus venosus (DV); Lower panel shows high pulsatility pattern in cases of severe IUGR indicating signs of cardiac failure (53-56). (*Right*): Upper panel shows the normal pulsatility of the middle cerebral artery in mid-gestation during morphogenesis (cephalization) of the fetal brain. Lower panel illustrates the Doppler pattern observed in fetus with IUGR (47-52).

(b) Doppler (Blood Flow) of Umbilical Cord (Vein and Artery)

Blood flow in the umbilical cord is significant by the 2nd trimester of pregnancy. Blood movement (pulsality) and flow (amount available to the fetus) via the umbilical vein and return from the fetus by umbilical artery can be assessed by pulse Doppler analysis. Placental blood with sufficient nutrients, O_2 and growth factors are essential for normal fetal development. Abnormalities in the blood flow are of importance in evaluating the etiology of IUGR and the prognosis (43-44). The parameters of blood transport by the pulse Doppler allow further evaluation of the IUGR and assessment of fetal well being (Figure 8). Since blood flows in the umbilical artery is toward the placenta, change in the placental function may be apparent in this flow. In a normal state, the placenta has a low resistance, and thus allow for a significant flow even during fetal diastole.

Placental pathology may lead to an increased resistance, for example, pathology due to features in the vasculature (narrow vessel diameter), thrombus formation or a decrease in the functional volume. In placental abruption, blood flow toward the placenta is reduced at time of diastole, leading to an absent end diastolic flow, and in more severe cases a reverse end diastolic flow may be observed. The Doppler patterns of the umbilical artery are of prognostic value for assessing the IUGR, since such anomalies may be associated with the increased fetal morbidity. Such Doppler analysis of IUGR may also reveal the developmental status of the fetus: constitutionally small, have normal growth potential or it is secondary to non-placental pathology.

(c) Doppler (Blood Flow) within Fetal Compartment

Optimal cerebral and liver blood flow is important to development of the fetus (47-56). Blood flow characteristics in these organs may be different from other fetal organs and extremities. Doppler blood flow parameters in these organs are significant for clinical evaluation of the IUGR. In impaired blood flow conditions (placental insufficiency), blood supply may be redistributed into these organs for a continued supply with reduced resistance exhibited by a decreased ratio of systolic to diastolic blood pressures. The blood flow may indicate the relative supply of O_2, nutrients and growth factors (e. g., IGFs) into the fetal organs. Availability of these elements may regulate the multiplication and differentiation of fetal primordial cells (neuroblast, osteoblast, myoblast). Reduced number of cells in organs will produce an aberrant or disproportionate growth or impaired cognitive function for neural tissues.

The possibility that an optimal blood flow in these organs is specifically related to development of normal neural, liver or other tissues, and in the absence dysmorphogenesis, is yet to be demonstrated. However, fetal cardiac abnormality such as congestive heart failure will impair the flow through the ductus venosus, which may result in an increased pulsatility and in the most severe cases reverse flow (corresponding to the atrial contraction). Abnormalities in the flow in the ductus venosus are associated with significant morbidity, such as neurological sequelae, and mortality; this condition may necessitate delivery depending of the gestational age of the fetus.

Simultaneous measurements of umbilical venous, fetal hepatic and ductus venosus blood flow during 2nd and 3rd trimesters may allow in-depth characterization of IUGR and other fetal disorders (51-52). Since the fetal liver by 2nd trimester may be a source of growth and growth regulatory factors and the fetal liver receives 70-80% of venous return from the placenta containing fetal growth requirements, including growth and regulatory factors generated by the placenta, normal development of fetal liver is essential to overall growth of the fetus. Therefore, such analysis of blood flow characteristics may define the overall organogenesis and development potential of the fetus *in utero*.

Uterine blood flow represents availability of maternal contributions, in particular, basic nutrients, endocrine factors and biochemical substrates to developing conceptus tissues for transfer into the fetal compartment. The significance of absence of impendence and loss of elasticity of the smooth muscle cells of the uterine spiral artery due to aggregation trophoblast cells in the endothelium of the arterial wall making it rigid and wider in diameter during pregnancy for continued delivery of oxygen and nutrients into placental-fetal complex, is unclear (2-3). This process ensures the availability of growth requirements for the fetus even at maternal costs and without maternal controls. However, uterine blood flow is considered as a predictor of pregnancy complications such as IUGR and preeclampsia (57).

3. Growth Factors of Conceptus Cells and Tissues

(a) Insulin Like Growth Factors (IGFs) during Prenatal and Postnatal Periods

A variety of growth factors and hormones are produced during development. Among the growth factors, IGF1 and -2 significantly influence the somatic growth (increase in cell number) and promote differentiation of cells. IGFs are synthesized both during the postnatal (children and adult) and prenatal (embryo-fetus-placenta) periods (58-60). During the postnatal period, IGF1 is produced by endocrine processes in the liver and production is regulated by the hypothalamic growth hormone releasing factor (GHRH) and growth hormone generated by the anterior pituitary (GH1; Figure 10; Left). *IGF1* gene has six exons (Figure 10; Right) which express variably with multiple transcription sites encoding for two IGF1 precursors: IGF1A and -1B. Biologically active IGF1 is a 76 amino acids (AA) peptide generated from exons 2 and 3 of the gene (61-65). *IGF1* protein in the plasma is transported to the target sites bound with IGF-binding proteins (BPs) (66-67).

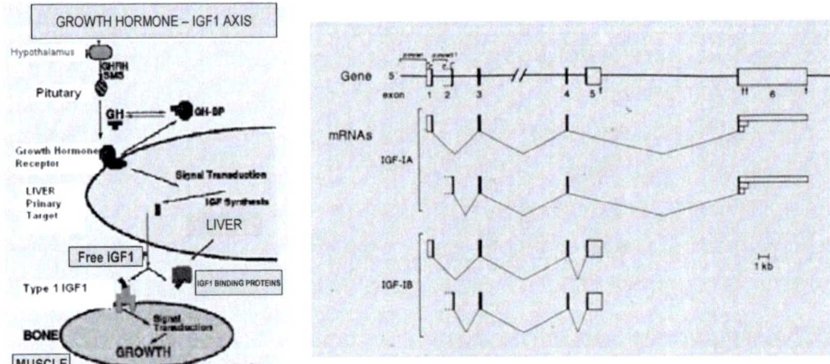

Left: GH-IGF1 Axis Right: IGF1 Gene Exons and Introns

Figure 10. Pictorials for GH-IGF axis during the postnatal periods (left) and two transcripts IGF1A and IGF1B (right). IGF is produced by the liver and regulated by pituitary GH during the postnatal period. IGFs are bound to BPs in plasma for delivery to target tissues (bone, muscle and neural). The IGF1 gene has six exons and introns and produces two transcripts, IGF1A and IGF1B.

However, in the prenatal period, the placenta is the primary source of IGFs and its regulatory factors. IGF1 and -2 are expressed in different cell types of human placenta as early as 6 weeks of gestation. They play a major role in the development and function of the placenta. IGF-1 promotes cell division (mitosis) and differentiation of diverse fetal tissues during pregnancy. The primary regulatory factors for IGFs biosynthesis in placenta are: a variant growth hormone (PGH [GH-2]; 68-76) and ghrelin (GHRL; 77-80) which is a releasing factor for the growth hormone generated by the human placenta.

In addition, multiple IGF-BPs are synthesized by the stromal cells of the chorionic villi, fetal membranes and basal plate (81-84). Placenta also produces a number of metalloproteinases (e. g., PAPP-A and ADAM-12s; 85-88). These metalloproteinases have been biochemically characterized as proteolytic enzymes (89-92). They decouple IGF-BPs releasing free IGFs (103-107). The free IGFs may bind to receptors promoting cell divisions in the fetus and placenta. PAPP-A is available in plasma as a complex of proform of major eosinophil basic protein (Pro-MBP) (108-110). The proteolytic property of PAPP-A is inhibited by Pro-MBP (105-110). It is suggested that autocrine-paracrine processes regulate biosynthesis of IGFs by GHRL and GH-2, and bioavailability of free IGFs from IGF-BP by metalloproteinase enzymes (PAPP-A and ADAM-12s) within the conceptus cells and tissues during human pregnancy.

The gene knockout studies in mice and other experimental studies have identified the vital roles of IGF axis in fetal and placental development showing that *igf1* affect the fetal and placental development; whereas, *igf2* enhances placental development and nutrient mobilization (111- 114). Absence of *igf-* and *igf-* receptor functions by targeted disruption is often lethal depending upon the background mice used. The phenotypic characteristics in gene disrupted mice may include marked hypoplasia of various organ and infertility. The severity of growth deficiency associated with the null mutations of *igf1* and *igf2* genes is as much as 60% of normal birth weight. These genes affect the morphogenesis of different fetal organs: muscle, bone, neural, gut, kidney and mammary gland. The biosynthesis and bioavailability of IGF- growth and regulatory factors in the anomalous human placenta, in particular that of IGF2 which is presumably related to placental growth and function, and the impact of placental anomalies and growth factor biosynthesis on fetal development during pregnancy remain unknown.

(b) Cellular Sources of Growth and Regulatory Factors during Pregnancy

IGFs and IGF-BPs are expressed in different cell types: cytotrophoblast and stroma of chorionic villi, fetal membranes and decidua (Table 1). The expression of these factors in the cytotrophoblast cells are reduced with further differentiation into multinucleated syncytiotrophoblast.

Table 1

Placental Factors	Cytotrophoblast (Villous/Extra-villous)	Syncytiotropho-blast (Multinucleated)	Villi stroma	References
IGFs /IGF-R	Yes	Yes	-	81,83,84
GHRL	Yes	Reduced	-	77,78
GH-2 (PGH)	Yes	-		71,72, 73
IGF-BPs	Yes (BP-3)	-	BP-3, - 4, -5	81,82, 83,102
PAPP-A ADAM-12s	Yes Yes	Reduced Yes	- ?	85,86, 87 88

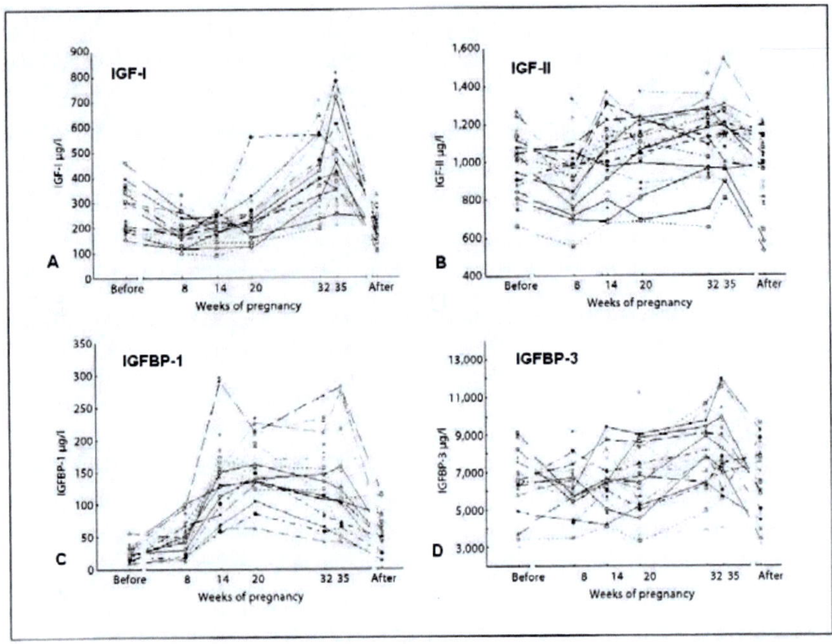

Figure 11. Concentrations of IGF1 and -2 and IGFBP1 and -3 in maternal sera during different weeks of normal pregnancy. These factors are produced abundantly and levels progressively increase during pregnancy and fall after delivery (116).

(c) Longitudinal Concentrations of IGFs, IGF-BPs and PGH in Pregnancy Sera

The concentrations of IGF-1, -2, and IGFBP-1, -3 in maternal sera are variable during pregnancies (115-116). IGF1 level initially decreases by 30%, while it increases by more than 50% compared to that before and end of the pregnancy (116). BP-3 is abundantly produced and carries 80-90% of the IGFs in plasma during pregnancy. The IGF and BP levels in the maternal sera are independent predictor and correlate with the IUGR, preterm and pre-eclampsia and fetal bone mass and body composition (117-121). The progressive changes in their levels during normal pregnancy are shown below (Figure 11).

PGH (GH2) is a variant growth hormone secreted by human placenta with differences in 12 amino acids from growth hormone (GH1) produced normally by the pituitary (122-125). The levels of PGH in the maternal sera increase progressively during pregnancy and they correlate with the gestational age, gender and disorders of pregnancy (Figure 12). Serum PGH concentration is significantly increased by mid-pregnancy in a normal pregnancy and a reduced level is an index of IUGR (126). The pituitary growth hormone (GH1) levels are reduced in maternal sera during pregnancy.

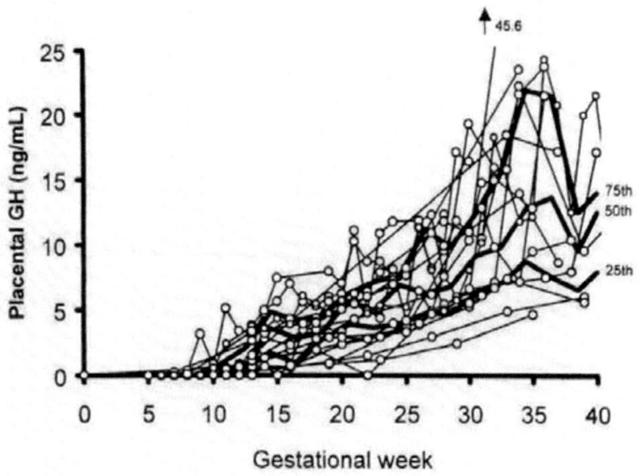

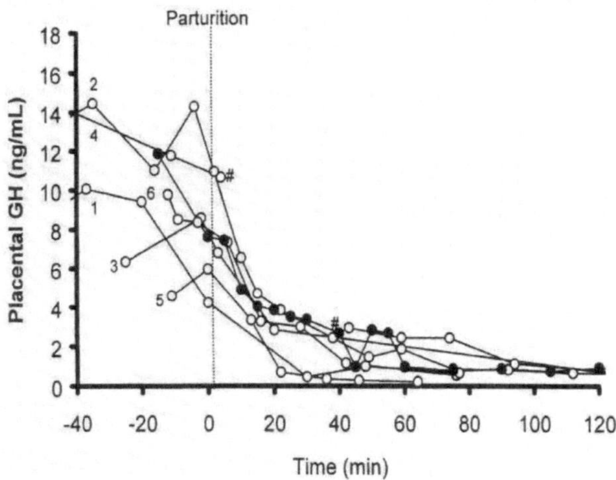

Figure 12. PGH concentrations during different periods of human normal pregnancy. It is secreted in significant amount in the maternal plasma by 1st trimester (7th week), achieves highest levels during the 3rd trimester (30-35 weeks), and reduced significantly after delivery. Consistent production reflects the normalcy of the pregnancy and the outcome (125).

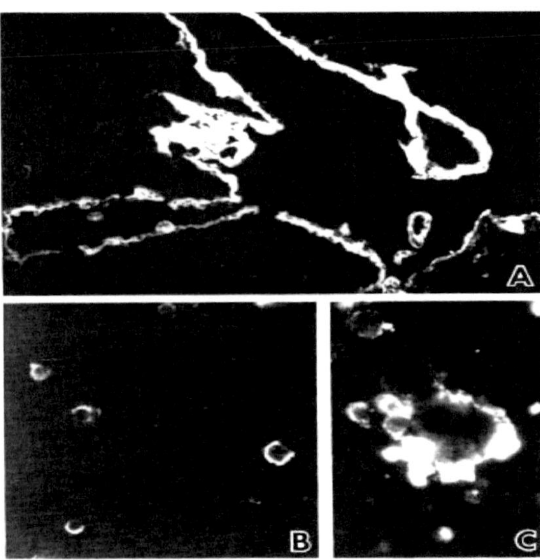

Figure 13. A (upper) - section of chorionic villi with fluorescent cytotrophoblast cell layer; B (lower, left) - isolated and purified trophoblast cells exhibiting expression of β-CG; C (lower, right) - clumps of cultured trophoblast cells (syncytiotrophoblast). X200. (86)

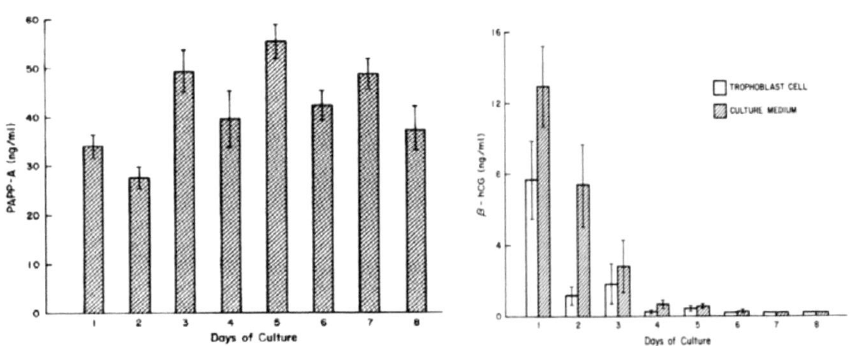

Left: Pregnancy Assoc. Plasma Protein (PAPP-A)

Right: β-hCG of the same culture Media

Figure 14. Biosynthesis and release of PAPP-A (left) and β-CG (right) by isolated and purified trophoblast cells in culture (86).

The PGH levels increase in maternal and fetal sera during preeclampsia and is also measurable in the amniotic fluid (127-128). The influence of PGH on IGF biosynthesis is of considerable interest as these factors are produced by the placental cells. Similarly, ghrelin (GHRL) is a growth hormone releasing factor and its role on the variant placental growth hormone (PGH; GH2) is unclear. It is likely, however, that auto- and paracrine processes regulate IGF biosynthesis in trophoblast cells involving: GHRL influencing PGH production and subsequently PGH promoting biosynthesis of IGF.

(d) Regulatory Factors for Bioavailability of IGFs

PAPP-A is a metalloproteinase produced by trophoblast cells (85-87) and PAPP-A is vital to fetal development (101). It is measurable in increasing concentration in the maternal blood with the progress of pregnancy and photolytic to IGFBP4 and IGFBP5 (95-96). Disintegrin metalloproteinases are another family of proteolytic enzymes (A Disintegrin and Metalloprotease 12; ADAM 12s) with activity toward IGFBP 3 and -5 is also generated during pregnancy (93-94). Both PAPP-A (129-135) and ADAM-12s (136-141) in maternal sera are also markers for other adverse human pregnancy conditions. In addition, these metalloproteinases may also have other functions during pregnancy, such as, immunosuppression and interaction with immune related antigens (major histocompatibility) which are as yet unclear (86).

The trophoblast cells can be isolated from first trimester chorionic villi and purified by centrifugation through a Ficoll-Hypaque gradient (86). Purified cytotrophoblast cells cultured in a tissue culture medium with bovine serum and antibiotics showed that PAPP-A and β-hCG are synthesized by such cells and released in the culture media. These cells expressed β-CG in such culture which can be localized by immunocytochemistry procedures confirming their trophoblast characteristics (Figure 13). These isolated cytotrophoblast cells aggregate in culture and a model for studies on studies on the factors regulate their differentiation. Concentrations of O_2 , bone morphogenetic factor-4 and cytokines are known to be regulators of trophoblast cell differentiation and function (88).

Gene knockout experiments for *papp-a* gene in mice have shown that it is an essential factor required for fetal development (101). PAPP-A is a metalloproteinase metzincin peptide of 1547 amino acids and the gene is of 22 exons with introns of variable sizes (89-92). PAPP-A is secreted as a 400 kDa dimer protein which binds covalently with proform-eosinophil major basic protein (500-kDa; pro-MBP) inhibiting the proteinase activity of PAPP-A (107). Nearly 99% of PAPP-A in pregnancy sera exists as an inactive complex bound with pro-MBP (108-109). The proteolytic activity of PAPP-A enzyme cleaves and releases IGFs bound with BPs (IGFBP4 and IGFBP5), and free IGFs then become available for cell division and differentiation of fetal and placental tissues (95-99). PAPP-A presumably acts as a local regulator of bioavailability of IGFs (102). The molecular regulatory processes for functions PAPP-A are outlined below (Figure 15, 107). The Pro-MBP subunit interacts with the proteolysis domain of PAPP-A inhibiting generation of active PAPP-A, essential for bioavailability of IGFs.

The biological activities of PAPP-A and other metalloproteinases are important for fetal growth and maintenance of human pregnancy (140-143). These factors may also provide immunosuppression for maintenance of pregnancy (86). Therefore, concentrations of these factors in the maternal sera may act as biomarkers even during the early gestation periods (first trimester) for fetal growth (IUGR) and other adverse pregnancy conditions of chromosomal anomalies (aneuploidy) and deleterious environmental maternal cigarette smoke exposure. Reduced concentrations of these factors in the maternal sera reflect sub-normal placental functions. Longitudinal measurement of PAPP-A and β-CG in maternal sera during pregnancy showed a progressive increase in their concentrations until delivery. Numerous studies on pregnancy have shown that reduced levels of metalloproteinases (PAPP-A and ADAM 12s) in maternal sera are associated with adverse pregnancy outcomes and fetal development.

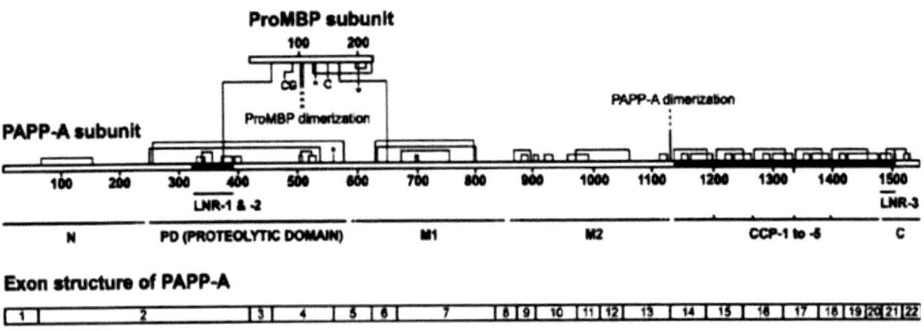

PAPP-A/Pro-MBP (Precursor Protein) => Free PAPP-A + MBP
(*Mechanisms are unknown*)
IGFs-BP + PAPP-A => Free IGF + BP
(*PAPP-A Catalyzes IGF release*)

Figure 15. PAPP-A and Pro-MBP Complex (upper) and PAAP-A Gene (Lower)

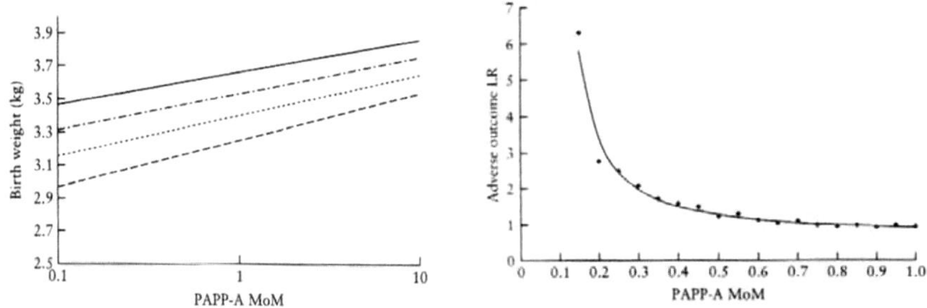

Figure 16. Correlation of reduced maternal serum levels of PAPP-A during different types of adverse pregnancy complications and birth weight. *Left:* PAPP-A values (MoM) of maternal sera correlate with the birth weight for pregnancies delivered at: 38 (- - - - -), 39 (……..), 40 (- . - . -) and 41 (____) weeks of normal gestation (140). *Right*: Best fit plot of PAPP-A concentration for preterm delivery (<37 week) and the likelihood ratio (LR). Regression in solid line and dots are individual data points (141).

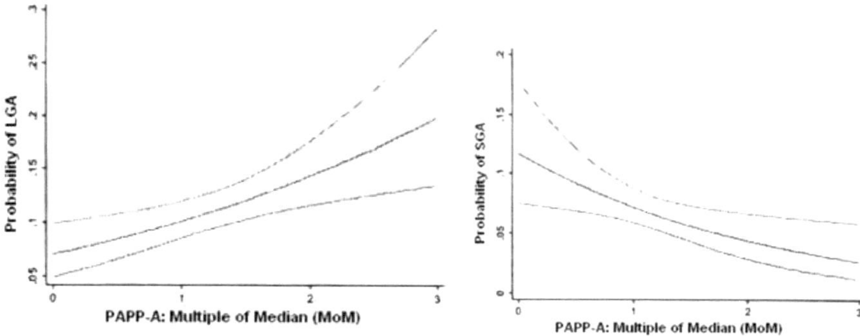

Figure 17. Logistic regression plot of maternal serum PAPP-A and probability of large-for-gestation (LGA; left) and small-for-gestation (SGA; right) (142). The regression line (middle) and upper and lower confidence intervals 5th and 95th limits are depicted.

A combination of ultrasound imaging of the fetus during first trimester of pregnancy and a reduced maternal serum levels of PAPP-A and β-CG identifies diverse fetal anomalies during the 1st and 2nd trimesters of pregnancy. The serum levels of PAPP-A and ADAM-2s expressed as Multiples of Median (MoM) of expected normal for a pregnancy of same gestational age may correlate with an adverse pregnancy outcome. These adverse pregnancy conditions are nuchal translucency and chromosome number, fetal growth retardation (IUGR), preeclampsia and deleterious effects of environmental exposure (129-146). Figure 16 illustrates the relationship of

PAPP-A concentrations in maternal sera to birth weight and preterm pregnancy (140-141). A lower PAPP-A concentration in the maternal sera correlate with reduced *in utero* fetal growth and shorter gestation periods in preterm pregnancy.

The probability estimates of fetal growth at birth: small-for-gestation (SGA) and large-for-gestation (LGA) rationalized for variability between samples is shown in Figure 17 (142). The fetal growth correlates with maternal sera PAPP-A concentrations (MoM) indicates its vital functions during pregnancy.

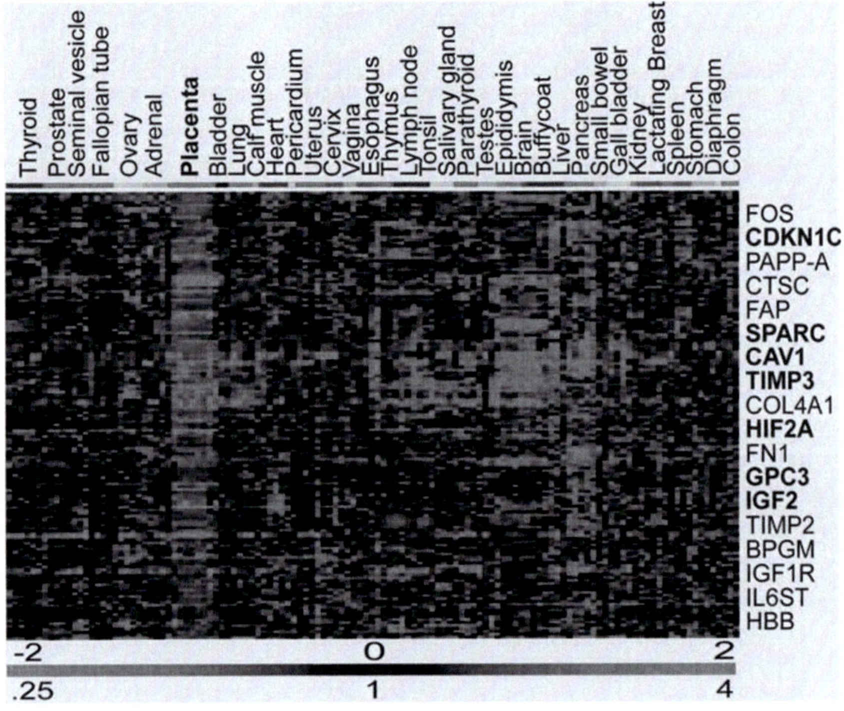

Figure 18. The microarray shows expression profile of different genes in villous parenchyma of normal term human placenta at delivery compared to other human tissues (154). A profile of genes (right side) and different tissues tested at the top. This two color microarray shows augmented expression (red) of placenta genes listed on the right side of the panel. Affymetrix microarray chips of oligonucleotides (70-mer) and 47,000 gene transcripts representing 24000 human genes (Human Genome U133 Plus 2.0) will allow a more detailed study (www.affymetrix.com/analysis/netaffx/showresults.affx).

(e) Umbilical Cord Blood Levels of Growth and Regulatory Factors

The vein of the umbilical cord is enrich with products generated by the maternal system and those from placental tissues; whereas, the two arteries of the umbilical cord bring nutrition and oxygen depleted blood from the fetus into the placenta. The umbilical cord blood concentrations of various growth and regulatory factors correlated with the birth weight and size of the neonate (147-151). These results confirm the assumption that such factors are indeed essential to fetal growth and development.

4. Expression of Placental Genes and Single Nucleotide Polymorphisms (SNPs)

(a) mRNA Expression in Placenta

Immunocytological studies of mRNA of specific genes have shown that placental cells are active (152-153). A recent innovation in this area is application of microarray chips for analysis of expression of multiple genes simultaneously. mRNA profiles of numerous genes correlate with the physiological state and pathology of the human placenta (154-157). The placental transcriptome was characterized by comparing the gene-expression patterns in samples from the villus parenchyma portions of placenta with 35 different tissue types (Figure 18; 154). A two-color approach with the same reference sample as a common internal standard in all hybridization for mRNA expression in normal placenta relative to other organs using the Affymetrix expression gene-chip revealed that some genes are preferentially expressed. The patterns of expression most abundant in placenta were analyzed by significance analysis method for microarrays showing expression levels were higher in placental villus parenchyma compared to other tissues. The significantly expressed genes were hierarchically clustered. Genes abundantly expressed in villus regions of placenta relative to other normal human tissues included IGF 2 and PAPPA which are known to be expressed in placenta. Altered expressions of specific genes (mRNA) correlate to the physiological or pathological states (155-157). These methods can be combined with the proteomic microarray assays or Western blotting for quantitation of protein biomarkers in biological samples to explore the molecular mechanisms related to their biosynthesis and regulation.

(b) Single Nucleotide Polymorphisms (SNPs) of IGFs and Regulatory Factors

SNPs are the most frequent type of variation characterized by the presence of alternative bases in the same site at frequencies greater than 1% in human population. Individual SNPs in a candidate gene are often ineffective in predicting disorders. However, frequent SNPs at the same site of the gene and haplotypes (collection of SNPs throughout the functional regions) have greater predictive power for adverse fetal and placental development. Information on the functions and association of these gene with human diseases can be found in the databases: SNP:GeneView, HuGE navigator and OMIM.

Table 2. Identified SNPs of Candidate Genes Associated with Pregnancy Disorders. and Fetal Development in the NCBI Database on SNPs.

Gene Name	SNP-Database	GENE
(Gene ID)	(www.ncbi.nlm.nih.gov/SNP/*link)	(All SNP)**
Insulin like Growth Factor IGF1 (3479)	*(snp_ref.cgi?locusId=3479)	109
Insulin like Growth Factor IGF2 (3481)	(snp_ref.cgi?locusId=3481) (snp3D.cgi?rsnum=1803647)	215
Insulin like Growth Factor Recep IGF1R (3480)	(snp_ref.cgi?locusId=3480); (snp3D.cgi?rsnum=17847196)	2518
Insulin like Growth Factor Bind Prot 3 IGFBP 3(3486)	(snp_ref.cgi?locusId=3486)	118
Insulin like Growth Factor Bind Prot 4 IGFBP 4(3487)	(snp_ref.cgi?locusId=3487); (snp3D.cgi?rsnum=35584955)	125
Pregnancy Assoc Plasma Prot PAPP-A (5069)	(snp_ref.cgi?locusId=5069); (snp3D.cgi?rsnum=3827668)	1312
A Disintegrin Metalloprotease 12 ADAM-12 (8038)	(snp_ref.cgi? locusId=8038) (snp3D.cgi?rsnum=2290843)	2761

** SNPs in these candidate genes, identified thus far, are in the GENE column. These sequence variations are synonymous, non synonymous or missense mutations and some of them are validated by different methods. Biological significance is also frequently listed in the website which is frequently revised as new data become available.

Some of the SNP of candidate genes (IGFs and regulatory factors) that may affect development and function of the fetus and placenta are in: www.ncbi.nlm.nih.gov/sites/gene (SNP database;Table 2).

Genomic alterations (deletions and SNPs) of the IGF1 gene have been shown to correlate with IUGR and to have effects during the postnatal development (158-162). SNPs in other candidate genes, in particular, IGF-receptor genes (IGFR1) have also been suggested to influence the intrauterine fetal growth and postnatal short stature of the individual (163-166). Mutations of the IGFR1 gene at different sites of the gene are associated with human fetal and postnatal growth (167-170). A case report of a point mutation of Arg108Gln/Lys115 Asn in a female and nonsense mutation of Arg59stop in the exon 2 of the *IGF1* receptor induced IUGR and poor postnatal growth (167). Mutation of the cleavage site (Arg-Lys-Arg-Arg) associated with processing of mature *IGF1R1* may produce resistance to *IGF1* and IUGR have been demonstrated (168). In addition, association of variation of genes for IGF2 and its receptor associated with fetal growth, and haplotypes of insulin and IGF2 level in umbilical cord blood have been shown. A recent study showing that PAPP-A gene and binding proteins may have SNP (171-172), their possible association of such SNPs with pregnancy disorders remains to be explored.

Conclusion

Fetal growth disorders *in utero* and premature births are major obstetrical problems. More than one half million (1 in 8) each year (http://www.cdc.gov/Features/PrematureBirth/) in the U. S. A. and more than 20 million of births worldwide (15.5%) are with low birth weight or premature for gestation periods (http://www.who.int/reproductive-health/publications/low_birthweight/). They are the leading cause of infant mortality and morbidity producing life long disabilities, including neural and cognitive deficits, blindness and numerous metabolic diseases (173-175). The cost of welfare of such children is more than 25 billion dollars in the U.S.A., ten times more than normal pregnancies. Analysis of fetal development, in particular, fetal organogenesis of the brain, liver, bone and muscle by the 3-D ultrasonographic imaging and blood flow patterns in placental and fetal compartments by pulse Doppler predicting the fetal and placental development and fetal well being during the pregnancy non-invasively is a significant advance. Physiological and molecular studies have shown that IGFs and their regulatory factors (GHRL, GH-2 and PAPP-A/ADAM-12s) are primarily generated by the placenta during human pregnancy. The biosynthesis and bioavailability of IGFs is regulated by autocrine and paracrine processes. Expression of genes and genomic variations studies of these genes may provide information on another dimension related to the genesis of these factors. These factors may act as biomarkers for various adverse pregnancies and further physiological, biochemical and genomic characterization of these factors will allow for precision diagnosis, intervention and therapy of disorders associated with the deficiency in their production and bioavailability. This review has provided an outline of an important direction for early diagnosis, intervention and possible therapy of such pregnancy disorders.

Acknowledgments

We gratefully appreciate the financial support of the National Institutes of Health over the years for our studies outlined in this review. One of us (M.K.S.) wishes to thank Dr. Mary D'Alton, Chair, Department of Obstetrics and Gynecology, Columbia University for providing excellent facilities and resources to develop the review at Columbia and also to Dr. Regina Santella for stimulating discussion and editing the manuscript.

References

[1] Patten, BM. *Human Embryology*, McGraw-Hill Book Co., New York, 1968

[2] Benirschke, K; Kaufman, P. Pathology of the Human Placenta. Placental shape aberrations 4th Edition, Springer Verlag, New York, NY 2000.

[3] Benirschke, K; Kaufman, P; Baergen, R. *The Human Placenta*. 5th Edition, Springer Verlag, New York, NY, 2006.

[4] Sanyal, MK; Li, YL; Belanger, K. Metabolism of polynuclear aromatic hydrocarbon in human placenta influenced by cigarette smoke exposure. *Reprod Toxicol*., 1994, 8, 411-418.

[5] Salafia, CM; Zhang, J; Miller, RK; Charles, AK; Shrout, P; Sun, W. Placental growth patterns affect birth weight for given placental weight. *Birth Defects Res A Clin Mol Teratol.*, 2007, 79, 281-8.

[6] Pardi, G; Cetin, I. Human fetal growth and organ development: 50 years of discoveries. *Am J Obstet Gynecol.*, 2006, 194, 1088-99.

[7] Hemachandra, AH; Klebanoff, MA. Use of serial ultrasound to identify periods of fetal growth restriction in relation to neonatal anthropometry. *Am J Hum Biol.*, 2006, 18, 791-7.

[8] Timor-Tritsch, IE; Monteagudo, A. Three and four-dimensional ultrasound in obstetrics and gynecology. *Curr Opin Obstet Gynecol.*, 2007, 19, 157-75.

[9] Kalache, KD; Bamberg, C; Proquitté, H; Sarioglu, N; Lebek, H; Esser, T. Three-dimensional multi-slice view: new prospects for evaluation of congenital anomalies in the fetus. *J Ultrasound Med.*, 2006, 25, 1041-9.

[10] Sonek, J. First trimester ultrasonography in screening and detection of fetal anomalies. *Am J Med Genet Semin Med Genet*, 2007, 145, 45-61.

[11] Yagel, S; Cohen, SM; Messing, B. First and early second trimester fetal heart screening. *Curr Opin Obstet Gynecol.*, 2007, 19, 183-90.

[12] Pilu, G; Segata, M; Ghi, T; Carletti, A; Perolo, A; Santini, D; Bonasoni, P; Tani, G; Rizzo, N. Diagnosis of midline anomalies of the fetal brain with the three-dimensional median view. *Ultrasound Obstet Gynecol.*, 2006, 27(5), 522-9.

[13] Boito, SM; Laudy, JA; Struijk, PC; Stijnen, T; Wladimiroff, JW. Three-dimensional US assessment of hepatic volume, head circumference, and abdominal circumference in healthy and growth-restricted fetuses. *Radiology*, 2002, 223, 661-5.

[14] Owen, P; Ogah, J; Bachmann, LM; Khan, KS. Prediction of intrauterine growth restriction with customised estimated fetal weight centiles. *BJOG.*, 2003, 110, 411-5.

[15] Ben-Haroush, A; Yogev, Y; Bar, J; Mashiach, R; Kaplan, B; Hod, M; Meizner, I. Accuracy of sonographically estimated fetal weight in 840 women with different pregnancy complications prior to induction of labor. *Ultrasound Obstet Gynecol.*, 2004, 23, 172-6.

[16] Chauhan, SP; Parker, D; Shields, D; Sanderson, M; Cole, JH; Scardo, JA. Sonographic estimate of birth weight among high-risk patients: feasibility and factors influencing accuracy. *Am J Obstet Gynecol.*, 2006, 195, 601-6.

[17] Chang, CH; Yu, CH; Chang, FM; Ko, HC; Chen, HY. The assessment of normal fetal liver volume by three-dimensional ultrasound. *Ultrasound Med Biol.*, 2003, 29, 1123-9.

[18] Chang, CH; Yu, CH; Ko, HC; Chen, CL; Chang, FM. Predicting fetal growth restriction with liver volume by three-dimensional ultrasound: efficacy evaluation. *Ultrasound Med Biol.*, 2006, 32, 13-7.

[19] Chang, CH; Yu, CH; Chang, FM; Ko, HC; Chen, HY. The assessment of normal fetal brain volume by 3-D ultrasound. *Ultrasound Med Biol.*, 2003, 29, 1267-72.

[20] Chang, CH; Chang, FM; Yu, CH; Ko, HC; Chen, HY. Three-dimensional ultrasound in the assessment of fetal cerebellar transverse and antero-posterior diameters. *Ultrasound Med Biol.*, 2000, 26, 175-82.

[21] Metzenbauer, M; Hafner, E; Hoefinger, D; Schuchter, K; Stangl, G; Ogris, E; Philipp, K. Three-dimensional ultrasound measurement of the placental volume in early pregnancy: method and correlation with biochemical placenta parameters. *Placenta*, 2001, 22, 602-605.

[22] Deurloo, K; Spreeuwenberg, M; Rekoert-Hollander, M; van Vugt, J. Reproducibility of 3-dimensional sonographic measurements of fetal and placental volume at gestational ages of 11-18 weeks. *J Clin Ultrasound.*, 2007, 35, 125-32.

[23] Abramowicz, JS; Sheiner, E. In utero imaging of the placenta: importance for diseases of pregnancy. *Placenta*, 2007, 28 Suppl A, S14-22.

[24] Baschat, AA; Güclü, S; Kush, ML; Gembruch, U; Weiner, CP; Harman, CR. Venous Doppler in the prediction of acid-base status of growth-restricted fetuses with elevated placental blood flow resistance. *Am J Obstet Gynecol.*, 2004, 191, 277-84.

[25] Botsis, D; Vrachnis, N; Christodoulakos, G. Doppler assessment of the intrauterine growth-restricted fetus. *Ann N Y Acad Sci.*, 2006, 1092, 297-303.

[26] Mari, G; Hanif, F; Treadwell, MC; Kruger, M. Gestational age at delivery and Doppler waveforms in very preterm intrauterine growth-restricted fetuses as predictors of perinatal mortality. *J Ultrasound Med.*, 2007, 26, 555-9.

[27] Turan, OM; Turan, S; Gungor, S; Berg, C; Moyano, D; Gembruch, U; Nicolaides, KH; Harman, CR; Baschat, AA. Progression of Doppler abnormalities in intrauterine growth restriction. *Ultrasound Obstet Gynecol.*, 2008, 2, 160-7.

[28] Hadlock, FP; Harrist, RB; Martinez-Poyer, J. In utero analysis of fetal growth: a sonographic weight standard. *Radiology*, 1991, 181, 129-33.

[29] Bernstein, IM; Mohs, G; Rucquoi, M; Badger, GJ. Case for hybrid "fetal growth curves": a population-based estimation of normal fetal size across gestational age. *J Matern Fetal Med.*, 1996, 5, 124-7.

[30] Fry, AG; Bernstein, IM; Badger, GJ. Comparison of fetal growth estimates based on birth weight and ultrasound references. *J Matern Fetal Neonatal Med.*, 2002, 12, 247-52.

[31] Reeves, S; Bernstein, IM. Optimal growth modeling. *Semin Perinatol.*, 2008, 32, 148-53.

[32] Gardosi, J; Chang, A; Kalyan, B; Sahota, D; Symonds, EM. Customised antenatal growth charts. *Lancet*, 1992, 339(8788), 283-7.

[33] Gardosi, J; Mongelli, M; Wilcox, M; Chang, A. An adjustable fetal weight standard. *Ultrasound Obstet Gynecol.*, 1995, 6, 168-74.

[34] Gardosi, J. Customized fetal growth standards: rationale and clinical application. *Semin Perinatol.*, 2004 Feb, 28, 33-40.

[35] Deter, RL. Individualized growth assessment: evaluation of growth using each fetus as its own control. *Semin Perinatol.*, 2004, 28, 23-32.

[36] Bernstein, IM; Goran, MI; Amini, SB; Catalano, PM. Differential growth of fetal tissues during the second half of pregnancy. *Am J Obstet Gynecol.*, 1997, 176, 28-32.

[37] Bernstein, IM; Plociennik, K; Stahle, S; Badger, GJ; Secker-Walker, R. Impact of maternal cigarette smoking on fetal growth and body composition. *Am J Obstet Gynecol.*, 2000, 183, 883-6.

[38] Bernstein, IM; Mongeon, JA; Badger, GJ; Solomon, L; Heil, SH; Higgins, ST. Maternal smoking and its association with birth weight. *Obstet Gynecol.*, 2005, 106, 986-91.

[39] Lee, W; Deter, RL; McNie, B; Gonçalves, LF; Espinoza, J; Chaiworapongsa, T; Romero, R. Individualized growth assessment of fetal soft tissue using fractional thigh volume. *Ultrasound Obstet Gynecol.*, 2004, 24, 766-74.

[40] Lee, W; Deter, RL; McNie, B; Gonçalves, LF; Espinoza, J; Chaiworapongsa, T; Balasubramaniam, M; Romero, R. The fetal arm: individualized growth assessment in normal pregnancies. *J Ultrasound Med.*, 2005, 24, 817-28.

[41] Lee, W; Deter, RL; Sameera, S; Espinoza, J; Gonçalves, LF; Romero, R. Individualized growth assessment of fetal thigh circumference using

three-dimensional ultrasonography. *Ultrasound Obstet Gynecol.*, 2008, 31, 520-8.

[42] Bornstein, R; Flores, AI; Montalban, MA; del Rey, MJ; de la Serna, J; Gilsanz, F. A modified cord blood collection method achieves sufficient cell levels for transplantation in most adult patients. *Stem Cells*, 2005, 23, 324-34.

[43] Viora, E; Sciarrone, A; Bastonero, S; Errante, G; Mortara, G; Chiappa, E; Campogrande, M. Anomalies of the fetal venous system: a report of 26 cases and review of the literature. *Fetal Diagn Ther.*, 2004, 19, 440-7.

[44] Rigano, S; Bozzo, M; Padoan, A; Mustoni, P; Bellotti, M; Galan, HL; Ferrazzi, E. Small size-specific umbilical vein diameter in severe growth restricted fetuses that die in utero. *Prenat Diagn.*, 2008 O, 28, 908-13.

[45] Schwarze, A; Gembruch, U; Krapp, M; Katalinic, A; Germer, U; Axt-Fliedner, R. Qualitative venous Doppler flow waveform analysis in preterm intrauterine growth-restricted fetuses with ARED flow in the umbilical artery--correlation with short-term outcome. *Ultrasound Obstet Gynecol.*, 2005, 25, 573-9.

[46] Hartung, J; Kalache, KD; Heyna, C; Heling, KS; Kuhlig, M; Wauer, R; Bollmann, R; Chaoui, R. Outcome of 60 neonates who had ARED flow prenatally compared with a matched control group of appropriate-for-gestational age preterm neonates. *Ultrasound Obstet Gynecol.*, 2005, 25, 566-72.

[47] Mari, G; Hanif, F; Kruger, M; Cosmi, E; Santolaya-Forgas, J; Treadwell, MC. Middle cerebral artery peak systolic velocity: a new Doppler parameter in the assessment of growth-restricted fetuses. *Ultrasound Obstet Gynecol.*, 2007, 29, 310-6.

[48] Hanif, F; Drennan, K; Mari, G. Variables that affect the middle cerebral artery peak systolic velocity in fetuses with anemia and intrauterine growth restriction. *Am J Perinatol.*, 2007, 24, 501-5.

[49] Ebbing, C; Rasmussen, S; Kiserud, T. Middle cerebral artery blood flow velocities and pulsatility index and the cerebroplacental pulsatility ratio: longitudinal reference ranges and terms for serial measurements. *Ultrasound Obstet Gynecol.*, 2007, 30, 287-96.

[50] Picklesimer, AH; Oepkes, D; Moise, KJ Jr; Kush, ML; Weiner, CP; Harman, CR; Baschat, AA. Determinants of the middle cerebral artery peak systolic velocity in the human fetus. *Am J Obstet Gynecol.*, 2007, 197, 526.e1-4.

[51] Fu, J; Olofsson, P. Fetal ductus venosus, middle cerebral artery and umbilical artery flow responses to uterine contractions in growth-restricted human pregnancies. *Ultrasound Obstet Gynecol.*, 2007, 30, 867-73.

[52] Mari, G; Hanif, F. Fetal Doppler: umbilical artery, middle cerebral artery, and venous system. *Semin Perinatol.*, 2008, 32, 253-7.

[53] Kiserud, T; Kessler, J; Ebbing, C; Rasmussen, S. Ductus venosus shunting in growth-restricted fetuses and the effect of umbilical circulatory compromise. *Ultrasound Obstet Gynecol.*, 2006, 28, 143-9.

[54] Bellotti, M; Pennati, G; De Gasperi, C; Bozzo, M; Battaglia, FC; Ferrazzi, E. Simultaneous measurements of umbilical venous, fetal hepatic, and ductus venosus blood flow in growth-restricted human fetuses. *Am J Obstet Gynecol.*, 2004, 190, 1347-58.

[55] Kessler, J; Rasmussen, S; Kiserud, T. The fetal portal vein: normal blood flow development during the second half of human pregnancy. *Ultrasound Obstet Gynecol.*, 2007, 30, 52-60.

[56] Kessler, J; Rasmussen, S; Godfrey, K; Hanson, M; Kiserud, T. Longitudinal study of umbilical and portal venous blood flow to the fetal liver: low pregnancy weight gain is associated with preferential supply to the fetal left liver lobe. *Pediatr Res.*, 2008, 63, 315-20.

[57] Dugoff, L; Lynch, AM; Cioffi-Ragan, D; Hobbins, JC; Schultz, LK; Malone, FD; D'Alton, ME. FASTER Trial Research Consortium.First trimester uterine artery Doppler abnormalities predict subsequent intrauterine growth restriction. *Am J Obstet Gynecol.*, 2005, 193(3 Pt 2), 1208-12.

[58] Rosenfeld, RG. Insulin-like growth factors and the basis of growth. *N Engl J Med.*, 2003, 349, 2184-6.

[59] Randhawa, R; Cohen, P. The role of the insulin-like growth factor system in prenatal growth. *Mol Genet Metab.*, 2005, 86, 84-90.

[60] Forbes, K; Westwood, M. The IGF axis and placental function. A mini review. *Horm Res.*, 2008, 69, 129-37.

[61] Rotwein, P; Pollock, KM; Didier, DK; Krivi, GG. Organization and sequence of the human insulin-like growth factor I gene. *J. Biol. Chem.*, 1986, 261, 4828-32.

[62] Kim, SW; Lajara, R; Rotwein, P. Structure and function of a human insulin-like growth factor 1 gene promoter. *Mol. Endocrin.*, 1992, 5, 1964-72.

[63] Jansen, E; Steenberg, PH; Leroith, D; Roberts, CT; Sussenbach, JS. Identification of multiple transcription start sites in the human insulin-like growth factor-I gene. *Mol. Cell. Endocrn.*, 1991, 78, 115-125.

[64] Sussenbach, JS; Steinbergh, PH; Holthuizen, P. Structure and expression of human insulin-like growth factor genes. *Growth Regulation.*, 1992, 2, 1-19.

[65] Steenberg, PH; Jansen, E; van Schaik, FMA; Sussenbach, JS. Functional analysis of the human IGF-I gene promoters. *Mol. Reprod. Devlop.*, 1993, 35, 365-367.

[66] Jones, JI; Clemmons, DR. Insulin-like growth factors and their binding proteins: biological actions. *Endocr Rev.*, 1995, 16, 3-34.

[67] Bach, LA; Headey, SJ; Norton, RS. IGF-binding proteins--the pieces are falling into place. *Trends Endocrinol Metab.*, 2005, 16, 228-34.

[68] Lacroix, MC; Guibourdenche, J; Frendo, JL; Muller, F; Evain-Brion, D. Human placental growth hormone- a review. *Placenta*, 2002, 23 Suppl A, S87-94.

[69] Handwerger, S; Freemark, M. The roles of placental growth hormone and placental lactogen in the regulation of human fetal growth and development. *J Pediatr Endocrinol Metab*, 2000, 13, 343-56.

[70] Seeburg, PH. The human growth hormone gene family: nucleotide sequences show recent divergence and predict a new polypeptide hormone. *DNA.*, 1982, 1, 239-49.

[71] MacLeod, JN; Lee, AK; Liebhaber, SA; Cooke, NE. Developmental control and alternative splicing of the placentally expressed transcripts from the human growth hormone gene cluster. *J Biol Chem.*, 1992, 267, 14219-26.

[72] Lacroix, MC; Guibourdenche, J; Fournier, T; Laurendeau, I; Igout, A; Goffin, V; Pantel, J; Tsatsaris, V; Evain-Brion, D. Stimulation of human trophoblast invasion by placental growth hormone. *Endocrino-logy*, 2005, 146, 2434-44.

[73] Fuglsang, J; Ovesen, P. Aspects of placental growth hormone physiology. *Growth Horm. IGF Res.*, 2006, 16, 67-85.

[74] Hu, L; Lytras, A; Bock, ME; Yuen, CK; Dodd, JG; Cattini, PA. Detection of placental growth hormone variant and chorionic somatomammotropin-L RNA expression in normal and diabetic pregnancy by reverse transcriptase-polymerase chain reaction. *Mol Cell Endocrinol.*, 1999, 157, 131-42.

[75] Caufriez, A; Frankenne, F; Hennen, G; Copinschi, G. Regulation of maternal IGF-I by placental GH in normal and abnormal human pregnancies. *Am J Physiol.*, 1993, 265(4 Pt 1), E572-7.

[76] Caufriez, A; Frankenne, F; Hennen, G; Copinschi, G. Regulation of maternal insulin-like growth factor I by placental growth hormone in pregnancy. Possible action of maternal IGF-I on fetal growth. *Horm Res.*, 1994, 42(1-2), 62-5.

[77] Gualillo, O; Caminos, J; Blanco, M; Garcìa-Caballero, T; Kojima, M; Kangawa, K; Dieguez, C; Casanueva, F. Ghrelin, a novel placental-derived hormone. *Endocrinology*, 2001, 142, 788-94.

[78] Bouhours-Nouet, N; Boux de Casson, F; Rouleau, S; Douay, O; Mathieu, E; Bouderlique, C; Gillard, P; Limal, JM; Descamps, P; Coutant, R. Maternal and cord blood ghrelin in the pregnancies of smoking mothers: possible markers of nutrient availability for the fetus. *Horm Res.*, 2006, 66, 6-12.

[79] Fuglsang, J; Skjaerbaek, C; Espelund, U; Frystyk, J; Fisker, S; Flyvbjerg, A; Ovesen, P. Ghrelin and its relationship to growth hormones during normal pregnancy. *Clin Endocrinol (Oxf).*, 2005, 62, 554-9.

[80] Lányi, E; Várnagy, A; Kovács, KA; Csermely, T; Szász, M; Szabó, I. Ghrelin and acyl ghrelin in preterm infants and maternal blood: relationship with endocrine and anthropometric measures. *Eur J Endocrinol.*, 2008, 158, 27-33.

[81] Hill, DJ; Clemmons, DR; Riley, SC; Bassett, N; Challis, JR. Immunohistochemical localization of insulin-like growth factors (IGFs) and IGF binding proteins -1, -2 and -3 in human placenta and fetal membranes. *Placenta*, 1993, 14, 1-12.

[82] Rogers, J; Wiltrout, L; Nanu, L; Fant, ME. Developmentally regulated expression of IGF binding protein-3 (IGFBP-3) in human placental fibroblasts: effect of exogenous IGFBP-3 on IGF-1 action. *Regul Pept.*, 1996, 61, 189-95.

[83] Han, VK; Bassett, N; Walton, J; Challis, JR. The expression of insulin-like growth factor (IGF) and IGF-binding protein (IGFBP) genes in the human placenta and membranes: evidence for IGF-IGFBP interactions at the feto-maternal interface. *J Clin Endocrinol Metab.*, 1996, 81, 2680-93.

[84] Shin, JC; Lee, JH; Yang, DE; Moon, HB; Rha, JG; Kim, SP. Expression of insulin-like growth factor-II and insulin-like growth factor binding

protein-1 in the placental basal plate from pre-eclamptic pregnancies. *Int J Gynaecol Obstet.*, 2003, 81, 273-80.

[85] Barnea, ER; Sanyal, MK; Brami, C; Bischof, P. In vitro production of pregnancy associated plasma protein-A (PAPP-A) by trophoblastic cells. *Arch Gynecol.*, 1986, 237, 187-190.

[86] Sanyal, MK; Brami, C; Bischof, P; Simmons, E; Barnea, ER; Dwyer, J; Naftolin, F. Immunoregulatory activity in supernatants from cultures of normal human trophoblast cells. *Am J Obstet Gynecol.*, 1989, 161, 446-453.

[87] Guibourdenche, J; Frendo, JL; Pidoux, G; Bertin, G; Luton, D; Muller, F; Porquet, D; Evain-Brion, D. Expression of pregnancy-associated plasma protein-A (PAPP-A) during human villous trophoblast differentiation in vitro. *Placenta*, 2003, 24, 532-9.

[88] Morrish, DW; Kudo, Y; Caniggia, I; Cross, J; Evain-Brion, D; Gasperowicz, M; Kokozidou, M; Leisser, C; Takahashi, K; Yoshimatsu, J. Growth factors and trophoblast differentiation--workshop report. *Placenta*, 2007, 28 Suppl A, S121-4.

[89] Kristensen, T; Oxvig, C; Sand, O; Moller, NP; Sottrup-Jensen, L. Amino acid sequence of human pregnancy-associated plasma protein-A derived from cloned cDNA. *Biochemistry*, 1994, 33, 1592-8.

[90] Laursen, LS; Overgaard, MT; Nielsen, CG; Boldt, HB; Hopmann, KH; Conover, CA; Sottrup-Jensen, L; Giudice, LC; Oxvig, C. Substrate specificity of the metalloproteinase pregnancy-associated plasma protein-A (PAPP-A) assessed by mutagenesis and analysis of synthetic peptides: substrate residues distant from the scissile bond are critical for proteolysis. *Biochem J.*, 2002, 367(Pt 1), 31-40.

[91] Boldt, HB; Kjaer-Sorensen, K; Overgaard, MT; Weyer, K; Poulsen, CB; Sottrup-Jensen, L; Conover, CA; Giudice, LC; Oxvig, C. The Lin12-notch repeats of pregnancy-associated plasma protein-A bind calcium and determine its proteolytic specificity. *J Biol Chem.*, 2004, 279, 38525-31.

[92] Boldt, HB; Overgaard, MT; Laursen, LS; Weyer, K; Sottrup-Jensen, L; Oxvig, C. Mutational analysis of the proteolytic domain of pregnancy-associated plasma protein-A (PAPP-A): classification as a metzincin. *Biochem J.*, 2001, 358(Pt 2), 359-67.

[93] Loechel, F; Fox, JW; Murphy, G; Albrechtsen, R; Wewer, UM. ADAM 12-S cleaves IGFBP-3 and IGFBP-5 and is inhibited by TIMP-3. *Biochem Biophys Res Commun.*, 2000, 278, 511-5.

[94] Shi, Z; Xu, W; Loechel, F; Wewer, UM; Murphy, LJ. ADAM 12, a disintegrin metalloprotease, interacts with insulin-like growth factor-binding protein-3. *J Biol Chem.*, 2000, 275, 18574-80.
[95] Lawrence, JB; Oxvig, C; Overgaard, MT; Sottrup-Jensen, L; Gleich, GJ; Hays, LG; Yates, JR 3rd; Conover, CA. The insulin-like growth factor (IGF)-dependent IGF binding protein-4 protease secreted by human fibroblasts is pregnancy-associated plasma protein-A. *Proc Natl Acad Sci (USA)*, 1999, 96, 3149-53.
[96] Laursen, LS; Overgaard, MT; Soe, R; Boldt, HB; Sottrup-Jensen, L; Giudice, LC; Conover, CA; Oxvig, C. Pregnancy-associated plasma protein-A (PAPP-A) cleaves insulin-like growth factor binding protein (IGFBP)-5 independent of IGF: implications for the mechanism of IGFBP-4 proteolysis by PAPP-A. *FEBS Lett.*, 2001, 504(1-2), 36-40.
[97] Laursen, LS; Overgaard, MT; Weyer, K; Boldt, HB; Ebbesen, P; Christiansen, M; Sottrup-Jensen, L; Giudice, LC; Oxvig, C. Cell surface targeting of pregnancy-associated plasma protein A proteolytic activity. Reversible adhesion is mediated by two neighboring short consensus repeats. *J Biol Chem.*, 2002, 277, 47225-34.
[98] Sun, IY; Overgaard, MT; Oxvig, C; Giudice, LC. Pregnancy-associated plasma protein A proteolytic activity is associated with the human placental trophoblast cell membrane. *J Clin Endocrinol Metab.*, 2002, 87, 5235-40.
[99] Overgaard, MT; Glerup, S; Boldt, HB; Rodacker, V; Olsen, IM; Christiansen, M; Sottrup-Jensen, L; Giudice, LC; Oxvig, C. Inhibition of proteolysis by the proform of eosinophil major basic protein (proMBP) requires covalent binding to its target proteinase. *FEBS Lett.*, 2004, 560, 147-52.
[100] Irwin, JC; Suen, LF; Cheng, BH; Martin, R; Cannon, P; Deal, CL; Giudice, LC. Human placental trophoblasts secrete a disintegrin metalloproteinase very similar to the insulin-like growth factor binding protein-3 protease in human pregnancy serum. *Endocrinology*, 2000, 141, 666-74.
[101] Conover, CA; Bale, LK; Overgaard, MT; Johnstone, EW; Laursen, UH; Fuchtbauer, EM; Oxvig, C; van Deursen, J. Metalloproteinase pregnancy-associated plasma protein A is a critical growth regulatory factor during fetal development. *Development*, 2004, 131, 1187-94.

[102] Boldt, HB; Conover, CA. Pregnancy-associated plasma protein-A (PAPP-A): a local regulator of IGF bioavailability through cleavage of IGFBPs. *Growth Horm IGF Res.*, 2007, 17, 10-8.

[103] Wasmoen, TL; McKean, DJ; Benirschke, K; Coulam, CB; Gleich, GJ. Evidence of eosinophil granule major basic protein in human placenta. *J Exp Med.*, 1989, 170, 2051-63.

[104] Wasmoen, TL; Coulam, CB; Benirschke, K; Gleich, GJ. Association of immunoreactive eosinophil major basic protein with placental septa and cysts. *Am J Obstet Gynecol.*, 1991, 165(2), 416-20.

[105] Plager, DA; Loegering, DA; Checkel, JL; Tang, J; Kephart, GM; Caffes, PL; Adolphson, CR; Ohnuki, LE; Gleich, GJ. Major basic protein homolog (MBP2): a specific human eosinophil marker. *J Immunol.*, 2006, 177, 7340-5.

[106] Plager, DA; Weiss, EA; Kephart, GM; Mocharla, RM; Matsumoto, R; Checkel, JL; Schwartz, LB; Gleich, GJ; Leiferman, KM. Identification of basophils by a mAb directed against pro-major basic protein 1. *J Allergy Clin Immunol.*, 2006, 117, 626-34.

[107] Overgaard, MT; Sorensen, ES; Stachowiak, D; Boldt, HB; Kristensen, L; Sottrup-Jensen, L; Oxvig, C. Complex of pregnancy-associated plasma protein-A and the proform of eosinophil major basic protein. Disulfide structure and carbohydrate attachment. *J Biol Chem.*, 2003, 278, 2106-17.

[108] Overgaard, MT; Haaning, J; Boldt, HB; Olsen, IM; Laursen, LS; Christiansen, M; Gleich, GJ; Sottrup-Jensen, L; Conover, CA; Oxvig, C. Expression of recombinant human pregnancy-associated plasma protein-A and identification of the proform of eosinophil major basic protein as its physiological inhibitor. *J Biol Chem.*, 2000, 275, 31128-33.

[109] Overgaard, MT; Glerup, S; Boldt, HB; Rodacker, V; Olsen, IM; Christiansen, M; Sottrup-Jensen, L; Giudice, LC; Oxvig, C. Inhibition of proteolysis by the proform of eosinophil major basic protein (proMBP) requires covalent binding to its target proteinase. *FEBS Lett.*, 2004, 560, 147-52.

[110] Glerup, S; Boldt, HB; Overgaard, MT; Sottrup-Jensen, L; Giudice, LC; Oxvig, C. Proteinase inhibition by proform of eosinophil major basic protein (pro-MBP) is a multistep process of intra- and intermolecular disulfide rearrangements. *J Biol Chem.*, 2005, 280, 9823-32.

[111] Baker, J; Liu, JP; Robertson, EJ. Efstratiadis A. Role of insulin-like growth factor in embryonic and postnatal growth. *Cell*, 1993, 75, 73-82.

[112] Allan, GJ; Flint, DJ; Patel, K. Insulin-like growth factor axis during embryonic development. *Reproduction*, 2001, 122, 31-9.

[113] Fowden, AL; Sibley, C; Reik, W; Constancia, M. Imprinted genes, placental development and fetal growth. *Horm Res.*, 2006, 65 Suppl 3, 50-8.

[114] Roberts, CT; Owens, JA; Sferruzzi-Perri, AN. Distinct actions of insulin-like growth factors (IGFs) on placental development and fetal growth: lessons from mice and guinea pigs. *Placenta*, 2008, 29 Suppl A, S42-7.

[115] Boyne, MS; Thame, M; Bennett, FI; Osmond, C; Miell, JP; Forrester, TE. The relationship of Insulin like growth factor (IGF-1), IGF binding proteins 1- and -2 and birth anthropometry: A prospective study. *J. Clin. Endocr. Metab.*, 2000, 88, 1687-91.

[116] Olausson, H; Lof, M; Brismar, K; Lewitt, M; Forsum, E; Sohlstrom, A. Longitudinal study of the maternal insulin-like growth factor system before, during and after pregnancy in relation to fetal and infant weight. *Horm Res.*, 69, 99-106, 2008.

[117] Leung, TY; Chan, LW; Leung, TN; Fung, TY; Sahota, DS; Lau, TK. First-trimester maternal serum levels of placental hormones are independent predictors of second-trimester fetal growth parameters. *Ultrasound Obstet Gynecol.*, 27, 156-61, 2006.

[118] Verhaeghe, J; Van Herck, E; Billen, J; Moerman, P; Van Assche, FA; Giudice, LC. Regulation of insulin-like growth factor-I and insulin-like growth factor binding protein-1 concentrations in preterm fetuses. *Am J Obstet Gynecol.*, 2003, 188, 485-91.

[119] Ingec, M; Gursoy, HG; Yildiz, L; Kumtepe, Y; Kadanali, S. Serum levels of insulin, IGF-1, and IGFBP-1 in pre-eclampsia and eclampsia. *Int J Gynaecol Obstet.*, 2004, 84, 214-9.

[120] Javaid, MK; Godfrey, KM; Taylor, P; Shore, SR; Breier, B; Arden, NK; Cooper, C. Umbilical venous IGF-1 concentration, neonatal bone mass, and body composition. *J Bone Miner Res.*, 2004, 19(1), 56-63.

[121] Akcakus, M; Koklu, E; Kurtoglu, S; Kula, M; Koklu, SS. The relationship among intrauterine growth, insulinlike growth factor I (IGF-I), IGF-binding protein-3, and bone mineral status in newborn infants. *Am J Perinatol.*, 2006, 23, 473-80.

[122] McIntyre, HD; Serek, R; Crane, DI; Veveris-Lowe, T; Parry, A; Johnson, S; Leung, KC; Ho, KK; Bougoussa, M; Hennen, G; Igout, A; Chan, FY; Cowley, D; Cotterill, A; Barnard, R. Placental growth

hormone (GH), GH-binding protein, and insulin-like growth factor axis in normal, growth-retarded, and diabetic pregnancies: correlations with fetal growth. *J Clin Endocrinol Metab.*, 2000, 85, 1143-50.

[123] Chellakooty, M; Skibsted, L; Skouby, SO; Andersson, AM; Petersen, JH; Main, KM; Skakkebaek, NE; Juul, A. Longitudinal study of serum placental GH in 455 normal pregnancies: correlation to gestational age, fetal gender, and weight. *J Clin Endocrinol Metab.*, 2002, 87, 2734-9.

[124] Chellakooty, M; Vangsgaard, K; Larsen, T; Scheike, T; Falck-Larsen, J; Legarth, J; Andersson, AM; Main, KM; Skakkebaek, NE; Juul, A. A longitudinal study of intrauterine growth and the placental growth hormone (GH)-insulin-like growth factor I axis in maternal circulation: association between placental GH and fetal growth. *J Clin Endocrinol Metab.*, 2004, 89, 384-91.

[125] Lønberg, U; Damm, P; Andersson, AM; Main, KM; Chellakooty, M; Lauenborg, J; Skakkebaek, NE; Juul, A. Increase in maternal placental growth hormone during pregnancy and disappearance during parturition in normal and growth hormone-deficient pregnancies. *Am J Obstet Gynecol.*, 2003, 188, 247-51.

[126] Papadopoulou, E; Sifakis, S; Giahnakis, E; Fragouli, Y; Karkavitsas, N; Koumantakis, E; Kalmanti, M. Increased human placental growth hormone at midtrimester pregnancies may be an index of intrauterine growth retardation related to preeclampsia. *Growth Horm IGF Res.*, 2006, 16, 290-6.

[127] Mittal, P; Espinoza, J; Hassan, S; Kusanovic, JP; Edwin, SS; Nien, JK; Gotsch, F; Than, NG; Erez, O; Mazaki-Tovi, S; Romero, R. Placental growth hormone is increased in the maternal and fetal serum of patients with preeclampsia. *J Matern Fetal Neonatal Med.*, 2007, 20, 651-9.

[128] Mittal, P; Hassan, SS; Espinoza, J; Kusanovic, JP; Edwin, S; Gotsch, F; Erez, O; Than, NG; Mazaki-Tovi, S; Romero, R. The effect of gestational age and labor on placental growth hormone in amniotic fluid. *Growth Horm IGF Res.*, 2008, 18, 174-9.

[129] Wapner, R; Thom, E; Simpson, JL; Pergament, E; Silver, R; Filkins, K; Platt, L; Mahoney, M; Johnson, A; Hogge, WA; Wilson, RD; Mohide, P; Hershey, D; Krantz, D; Zachary, J; Snijders, R; Greene, N; Sabbagha, R; MacGregor, S; Hill, L; Gagnon, A; Hallahan, T; Jackson, L. First Trimester Maternal Serum Biochemistry and Fetal Nuchal Translucency Screening (BUN) Study Group. First-trimester screening for trisomies 21 and 18. *N Engl J Med.*, 2003, 349, 1405-13.

[130] Malone, FD; Canick, JA; Ball, RH; Nyberg, DA; Comstock, CH; Bukowski, R; Berkowitz, RL; Gross, SJ; Dugoff, L; Craigo, SD; Timor-Tritsch, IE; Carr, SR; Wolfe, HM; Dukes, K; Bianchi, DW; Rudnicka, AR; Hackshaw, AK; Lambert-Messerlian, G; Wald, NJ; D'Alton, ME. First- and Second-Trimester Evaluation of Risk (FASTER) Research Consortium. First-trimester or second-trimester screening, or both, for Down's syndrome. *N Engl J Med.*, 2005, 353, 2001-2011.

[131] Nicolaides, KH; Spencer, K; Avgidou, K; Faiola, S; Falcon, O. Multicenter study of first-trimester screening for trisomy 21 in 75 821 pregnancies: results and estimation of the potential impact of individual risk-orientated two-stage first-trimester screening. *Ultrasound Obstet Gynecol.*, 2005, 25, 221-226.

[132] Smith, GC; Stenhouse, EJ; Crossley, JA; Aitken, DA; Cameron, AD; Connor, JM. Early pregnancy levels of pregnancy-associated plasma protein A and the risk of intrauterine growth restriction, premature birth, preeclampsia, and stillbirth. *J Clin Endocrinol Metab.*, 2002, 87, 1762-1767.

[133] Pilalis, A; Souka, AP; Antsaklis, P; Daskalakis, G; Papantoniou, N; Mesogitis, S; Antsaklis, A. Screening for pre-eclampsia and fetal growth restriction by uterine artery Doppler and PAPP-A at 11-14 weeks' gestation. *Ultrasound Obstet Gynecol.*, 2007, 29, 135-40.

[134] Spencer, K; Cowans, NJ; Nicolaides, KH. Low levels of maternal serum PAPP-A in the first trimester and the risk of pre-eclampsia. *Prenat Diagn.*, 2008, 28, 7-10.

[135] Ardawi, MS; Nasrat, HA; Rouzi, AA; Qari, MH; Al-Qahtani, MH; Abuzenadah, AM. Maternal serum free-beta-chorionic gonadotrophin, pregnancy-associated plasma protein-A and fetal nuchal translucency thickness at 10-13(+6) weeks in relation to co-variables in pregnant Saudi women. *Prenat Diagn.*, 2007, 27, 303-11.

[136] Christiansen, M; Spencer, K; Laigaard, J; Cowans, NJ; Larsen, SO; Wewer, UM. ADAM 12 as a second-trimester maternal serum marker in screening for Down syndrome. *Prenat Diagn.*, 2007, 27, 611-615.

[137] Spencer, K; Vereecken, A; Cowans, NJ. Maternal serum ADAM12s as a potential marker of trisomy 21 prior to 10 weeks of gestation. *Prenat Diagn.*, 2008, 28, 209-211.

[138] Poon, LC; Chelemen, T; Granvillano, O; Pandeva, I; Nicolaides, KH. First-Trimester Maternal Serum a Disintegrin and Metalloprotease 12

(ADAM12) and Adverse Pregnancy Outcome. *Obstet Gynecol.*, 2008, 112, 1082-90.

[139] Spencer, K; Cowans, NJ; Stamatopoulou, A. ADAM12s in maternal serum as a potential marker of pre-eclampsia. *Prenat Diagn.*, 2008, 28, 212-216.

[140] Spencer, K; Cowans, NJ; Avgidou, K; Molina, F; Nicolaides, KH. First-trimester biochemical markers of aneuploidy and the prediction of small-for-gestational age fetuses. *Ultrasound Obstet Gynecol.*, 2008, 31, 15-9.

[141] Spencer, K; Cowans, NJ; Molina, F; Kagan, KO; Nicolaides, KH. First-trimester ultrasound and biochemical markers of aneuploidy and the prediction of preterm or early preterm delivery. *Ultrasound Obstet Gynecol.*, 2008, 31, 147-52.

[142] Peterson, SE; Simhan, HN. First-trimester pregnancy-associated plasma protein A and subsequent abnormalities of fetal growth. *Am J Obstet Gynecol.*, 2008, 198, e43-5.

[143] Cowans, NJ; Spencer, K. First-trimester ADAM12 and PAPP-A as markers for intrauterine fetal growth restriction through their roles in the insulin-like growth factor system. *Prenat Diagn.*, 2007, 27, 264-71.

[144] Leung, TY; Sahota, DS; Chan, LW; Law, LW; Fung, TY; Leung, TN; Lau, TK. Prediction of birth weight by fetal crown-rump length and maternal serum levels of pregnancy-associated plasma protein-A in the first trimester. *Ultrasound Obstet Gynecol.*, 2008, 31, 10-4.

[145] Kagan, KO; Frisova, V; Nicolaides, KH; Spencer, K. Dose dependency between cigarette consumption and reduced maternal serum PAPP-A levels at 11-13+6 weeks of gestation. *Prenat Diagn.*, 2007, 27, 849-53.

[146] Pringle, PJ; Geary, MP; Rodeck, CH; Kingdom, JC; Kayamba-Kay's, S; Hindmarsh, PC. The influence of cigarette smoking on antenatal growth, birth size, and the insulin-like growth factor axis. *J Clin Endocrinol Metab.*, 2005, 90, 2556-62.

[147] Ostlund, E; Bang, P; Hagenas, L; Fried, G. Insulin-like growth factor 1 in fetal serum obtained by codocentesis is correlated with intrauterine growth retardation. *Hum. Reprod.*, 1997, 12, 840-4.

[148] Klauwer, D; Blum, WF; Hanitsch, S; Rascher, W; Lee, PD; Kiess, W. IGF-I, IGF-II, free IGF-I and IGFBP-1, -2 and -3 levels in venous cord blood: relationship to birth weight, length and gestational age in healthy newborns. *Acta Paediatr.*, 1997, 86, 826-33.

[149] Ong, K; Kratzsch, J; Kiess, W; Costello, M; Scott, C; Dunger, D. Size at birth and cord blood levels of insulin, insulin-like growth factor I (IGF-I), IGF-II, IGF-binding protein-1 (IGFBP-1), IGFBP-3, and the soluble IGF-II/mannose-6-phosphate receptor in term human infants. The ALSPAC Study Team. Avon Longitudinal Study of Pregnancy and Childhood. *J Clin Endocrinol Metab.*, 2000, 85, 4266-9.

[150] Fant, M; Salafia, C; Baxter, RC; et. al., Circulating level IGFs and IGF binding proteins in human cord serum relationships to intrauterine growth. *Reg. Protein*, 1993, 48, 29-30.

[151] Chanoine, JP; Yeung, LP; Wong, AC; Birmingham, CL. Immunoreactive ghrelin in human cord blood: relation to anthropometry, leptin, and growth hormone. *J Pediatr Gastroenterol Nutr.*, 2002, 35, 282-6.

[152] Sheikh, S; Satoskar, P; Bhartiya, D. Expression of insulin-like growth factor-I and placental growth hormone mRNA in placentae: a comparison between normal and intrauterine growth retardation pregnancies. *Mol Hum Reprod.*, 2001, 7, 287-92.

[153] Han, VK; Carter, AM. Spatial and temporal patterns of expression of messenger RNA for insulin-likegrowth factors and their binding proteins in the placenta of man and laboratory animals. *Placenta*, 2000, 21, 289-305.

[154] Sood, R; Zehnder, JL; Druzin, ML; Brown, PO. Gene expression patterns in human placenta. *Proc Natl Acad Sci*, USA., 2006, 103, 5478-83.

[155] Sitras, V; Paulssen, RH; Grønaas, H; Vårtun, A; Acharya, G. Gene expression profile in labouring and non-labouring human placenta near term. *Mol Hum Reprod.*, Epub 2007, 14, 61-5.

[156] Huuskonen, P; Storvik, M; Reinisalo, M; Honkakoski, P; Rysä, J; Hakkola, J; Pasanen, M. Microarray analysis of the global alterations in the gene expression in the placentas from cigarette-smoking mothers. *Clin Pharmacol Ther.*, 2008, 83, 542-50.

[157] Kang, BY; Tsoi, S; Zhu, S; Su, S; Kay, HH. Differential gene expression profiling in HELLP syndrome placentas. *Reprod Sci.*, 2008, 15, 285-94.

[158] Woods, KA; Camacho-Hubner, C; Savage, MO; Clark, AJ. Intrauterine growth retardation and postnatal failure associated with deletion of the insulin-like growth factor 1 gene. *N. Engl. J. Med.*, 1996, 335, 1363-7.

[159] Woods, KA; Camancho-Hubner, C; Barter, D; et al. Insulin-like growth factor 1 gene deletion causing intrauterine growth retardation and severe short stature. *Acta Paediatrica (Suppl).*, 1997, 423, 39-45.

[160] Camacho-Hubner, C; Woods, KA; Clark, AJ; Savage, MO. Insulin like growth factor (IGF)-1 gene deletion. *Endocr. Metab. Disorder*, 2002, 3, 357-61.

[161] Arends, N; Johnston, L; Hokken-Koelega, A; Van Duijn, C; De Ridder, M; Savage, M; Clark, A. Polymorphism in the IGF-I gene: clinical relevance for short children born small for gestational age (SGA). *J. Clin. Endocr. Metab.*, 2002, 87, 2720-4.

[162] Vaessen, N; Janssen, JA; Heutink, P; Hofman, A; Lamberts, SW; Oostra, BA; Pols, HA; van Duijn, CM. Association between genetic variation in the gene for insulin-like growth factor-1 and low birth weight. *Lancet*, 2002, 359, 1036-7.

[163] Kiess, W; Kratzsch, J; Keller, E; Schneider, A; Raile, K; Klammt, J; Seidel, B; Garten, A; Schmidt, H; Pfäffle, R. Clinical Examples of Disturbed IGF Signaling: Intrauterine and Postnatal Growth Retardation due to Mutations of the Insulin-Like Growth Factor I Receptor (IGF-IR) Gene. *Reviews in Endocrine & Metabolic Disorders*, 2005, 6, 183-187.

[164] Abuzzahab, MJ; Schneider, A; Goddard, A; Grigorescu, F; Lautier, C; Keller, E; Kiess, W; Klammt, J; Kratzsch, J; Osgood, D; Pfäffle, R; Raile, K; Seidel, B; Smith, RJ; Chernausek, SD. Intrauterine Growth Retardation (IUGR) Study Group.IGF-I Receptor Mutations Resulting in Intrauterine and Postnatal Growth Retardation. *N Engl J Med.*, 2003, 349, 2211-22.

[165] Walenkamp, MJ; van der Kamp, HJ; Pereira, AM; Kant, SG; van Duyvenvoorde, HA; Kruithof, MF; Breuning, MH; Romijn, JA; Karperien, M; Wit, JM. A Variable Degree of Intrauterine and Postnatal Growth Retardation in a Family with a Missense Mutation in the Insulin-Like Growth Factor I Receptor. *J Clin Endocrinol Metab.*, 2006, 91, 3062-3070.Inagaki, K; Tiulpakov, A; Rubtsov, P; Sverdlova, P; Peterkova, V; Yakar, S; Terekhov, S; LeRoith, D. A Familial Insulin-Like Growth Factor-I Receptor Mutant Leads to Short Stature: Clinical and Biochemical Characterization. *J Clin Endocrinol Metab*, 2007, 92, 1542-1548.

[167] Raile, K; Klammt, J; Schneider, A; Keller, A; Laue, S; Smith, R; Pfäffle, R; Kratzsch, J; Keller, E; Kiess, W. Clinical and Functional Characteristics of the Human Arg59Ter Insulin-Like Growth Factor I

Receptor (IGF1R) Mutation: Implications for a Gene Dosage Effect of the Human IGF1R. *J Clin Endocrinol Metab*, 2006, 91, 2264-2271.

[168] Kawashima, Y; Kanzaki, S; Yang, F; Kinoshita, T; Hanaki, K; Nagaishi, J; Ohtsuka, Y; Hisatome, I; Ninomoya, H; Nanba, E; Fukushima, T; Takahashi, S. Mutation at Cleavage Site of Insulin-Like Growth Factor Receptor in a Short-Stature Child Born with Intrauterine Growth Retardation. *J Clin Endocrinol Metab*, 2005, 90, 4679-4687.

[169] Kaku, K; Osada, H; Seki, K; Sekiya, S. Insulin-like growth factor 2 (IGF2) and IGF2 receptor gene variants are associated with fetal growth. *Acta Paediatr.*, 2007, 96, 363-7.

[170] Adkins, RM; Fain, JN; Krushkal, J; Klauser, CK; Magann, EF; Morrison, JC. Association between paternally Inherited Haplotypes upstream of the Insulin gene and umbilical cord IGF-II levels. *Pediatr Res.*, 2007 Jul 24; Publish Ahead of Print [Epub ahead of print]

[171] Canzian, F; McKay, JD; Cleveland, RJ; Dossus, L; Biessy, C; Rinaldi, S; Landi, S; Boillot, C; et. al., Polymorphisms of genes coding for insulin-like growth factor 1 and its major binding proteins, circulating levels of IGF-I and IGFBP-3 and breast cancer risk: results from the EPIC study. *Br J Cancer.*, 2006, 94, 299-307.

[172] Park, S; Youn, JC; Shin, DJ; Park, CM; Kim, JS; Ko, YG; Choi, D; Ha, JW; Jang, Y; Chung, N. Genetic polymorphism in the pregnancy-associated plasma protein-A associated with acute myocardial infarction. *Coron Artery Dis.*, 2007, 18, 417-22.

[173] Kok, JH; den Ouden, AL; Verloove-Vanhorick, SP; Brand, R. Outcome of very preterm small for gestational age infants: the first nine years of life. *Br J Obstet Gynaecol.*, 1998, 105, 162-8.

[174] Aucott, SW; Donohue, PK; Northington, FJ. Increased morbidity in severe early intrauterine growth restriction. *J Perinatol.*, 2004, 24, 435-40.

[175] Garite, TJ; Clark, R; Thorp, JA. Intrauterine growth restriction increases morbidity and mortality among premature neonates. *Am J Obstet Gynecol.*, 2004, 191, 481-7.

In: Human Placenta: Structure and Development... ISBN: 978-1-60876-457-0
Editors: E. Berven, et al. pp. 125-143 © 2010 Nova Science Publishers, Inc.

Chapter IV

Pregnancy-Specific Beta-1-Glycoproteins (PSGs): Structure, Functions and Biologically Active Peptides

Alexander A. Terentiev[*], *Innokenty M. Mokhosoev* *and Nurbubu T. Moldogazieva*
Department of Biochemistry, Russian State Medical University, Ostrovityanova Street, 1, Moscow, Russia.

Abstract

Pregnancy-specific glycoproteins (PSGs) are secreted proteins which are produced by the rodent and primate placenta and play a critical role in pregnancy success. Genes which encode PSGs belong to carcinoembryonic antigen (CEA) gene family, which is included in immunoglobulin (Ig) gene superfamily. In humans, to date there are 11 protein products of these genes which are designated as PSG1−11. In rodents there are 17 PSGs, which are designated as PSG16−32. Human PSGs were first discovered in serum of pregnant women and were initially named as trophoblast-specific beta globulins (TBGs). Little later they were isolated from placental extracts and also revealed in serum of patients with trophoblastic tumors. Biological role of PSGs is not fully

[*] Corresponding author: E-mail: aaterent@mtu-net.ru

elucidated to date. However a number of experimental data and clinical observations allow supposing their critical role in the maintenance of pregnancy. Low PSG levels in the maternal circulation are associated with threatened abortions, intrauterine retardation and fetal hypoxia.

It has been shown that PSGs function as immunomodulatory proteins which regulate activity of T-lymphocytes and secretion of cytokines by monocytes and macrophages. Also, PGSs may participate in maternal vasculature remodeling through influencing on secretion of pro-angiogenic agents such as transforming growth factor-beta-1 (TGF-β1) and vascular endothelial growth factor (VEGF) by different cell types involved in the development of placenta.

Several functional domains have been described in PSG structures. For example, tripeptide RGD has been revealed in N-terminal immunoglobulin (Ig)-like domain of most of human PSGs. It is proposed that RGD motif of PSGs is involved in binding to integrin receptors. Binding of mouse PSGs to integrin-associated receptor CD9 has been demonstrated. In our laboratory some human PSG-derived oligopeptide fragments have been shown to possess biological activity. This chapter is devoted to summarizing and analyzing of data on structure and function of PSGs known to date. Also, relatively recent data of PSG-derived biologically active peptides are described.

Introduction

Placenta is an essential organ for mammalian reproduction that links maternal and fetal compartments. To date a number of placenta-specific genes, enhancer elements and gene isoforms as well as placenta-specific members of gene families have been identified. Notably, there are two restrictions in placenta genes expression. First, not all of these genes are present in all placental mammals. Second, a very limited number of the genes are expressed in placenta [1, 2].

Genes, which encode pregnancy-specific glycoproteins (PSGs), are expressed almost exclusively in trophoblasts of haemochorial placenta of primates and rodents. Haemochorial placentation is a unique physiological process in which the fetal trophoblast cells remodel the maternal decidual spiral arteries to establish the fetoplacental blood supply [3−5].

The PSG subfamily of glycoproteins belongs to the carcinoembryonic antigen (CEA) family, which also includes the CEA-related cell adhesion molecules (CEACAMs). The CEA family is itself part of the immunoglobulin

(Ig) superfamily [6]. PSGs and some CEACAMs are expressed almost exclusively in trophoblasts suggesting potential functional convergence between these otherwise divergent gene subfamilies [7].

In humans the PSG proteins are encoded by at least 11 different genes clustered on chromosome 19q13.2, that give rise to 30 different proteins (including isoforms) through alternatively spliced mRNAs [8–10]. Seventeen mouse Psg genes are located on chromosome 7 [11]. Protein products of all above mentioned genes are designated as PSG1–11 in humans and as PSG16–32 in rodents.

It has been suggested that human and rodent Psg multigene families evolved independently via further gene duplication and exon shuffling events [12]. However, a semi-quantitative study of Psg gene expression in mouse pregnancy indicated that different family members exhibit different expression levels between E11 and E18, suggesting the possibility of divergent functions, at least within the mouse Psg family [11].

The PSGs are synthesized in the syncytiotrophoblast of human placenta and in the giant cells and spongiotrophoblast of rodent placenta [3–5, 13]. Also, human PSG1 can be detected as early as in the culture of pre-implantation human embryos [14]. Recently, it was demonstrated that human spermatozoa can deliver PSG1 mRNA to oocytes and the PSG1 transcript remained detectable for at least 24 hours after zygotic development [15]. PSG1 mRNA presents in spermatozoa of fertile men at higher levels than in infertile men. Taking into account that the protein product of Psg1 gene was not detected in sperm extracts, it could be postulated that its mRNA may be translated de novo in the newly formed zygote. Therefore, PSG1 may play a critical role in early embryo development and implantation.

Also, it has been demonstrated that mouse PSG proteins may be synthesized not only in placenta, but also in other tissues. PSG16 may be expressed in the brain and PSG18 is expressed in follicle-associated epithelium in the gut, where it may modulate immune response [16, 17].

Human pregnancy-specific beta-1-glycoprotein-1 was first discovered in 1970 by Yu.S. Tatarinov and V.N. Masyukevich [18] in serum of pregnant women and was initially named as trophoblast-specific beta-globulin (TBG). Little later it was isolated from placental extracts [19] and also was revealed in serum of patients with trophoblastic tumors [20].

In maternal circulation PSGs are detected as early as 7 days post-implantation [21]. During normal pregnancy, PSG molecules are released to maternal blood reaching 200–400 mkg/ml in serum at the end of gestation, far exceeding concentrations of human chorionic gonadotropin and alpha-fetoprotein (AFP) [21, 22]. In fetal serum PSG level does not exceed 1–2 mkg/ml.

During mammalian pregnancy the interaction between maternal uterine tissues and fetal trophoblasts is regulated by a wide variety of cellular and endocrinological mechanisms. These mechanisms provide trophoblastic invasion and remodelling of maternal tissues, placental angiogenesis, and modulation of maternal immune responses. Central to these processes is production by trophoblasts a variety of hormones that are found in abundance in the maternal bloodstream during pregnancy [23].

Low PSG levels are associated with certain pathological conditions during pregnancy. Specifically, low PSG levels in human maternal circulation are associated with threatened abortions, intrauterine growth retardation and fetal hypoxia [24]. Application of anti-PSG antibodies or vaccination with PSG induces abortion in mice and monkeys, and reduces fertility of non-pregnant monkeys [22, 25]. In addition, PSG-mediated suppression of T cells is correlated with increased maternal morbidity in purulent septic complications of abortion [26], and elevated circulating PSG levels are correlated with improved symptoms of rheumatoid arthritis [27].

Structure of PSGs

Structurally, PSGs are glycoproteins with molecular weight of its polypeptide chain from about 37 to 49 kDa in humans and from 44 to 54 kDa in rodents. Content of carbohydrate moiety of PSGs may vary from about 21 to 32% of total molecular weight. So, together with carbohydrates the total molecular weight of PSGs may constitute up to 72 kDa.

There may be from 3 to 8 glycolysation sites in different human PSGs (see Table 1). Interestingly, the consensus amino acid sequence for potential N-glycosylation sites is NXT/S, where X is any amino acid except proline [11]. Carbohydrate moieties may include galactose, mannose, fucose, N-acetylglucosamine and neuraminic acid.

Spatial structure of PSG molecules may be stabilized by disulphide bridges. PSG molecules contain from 5 (PSG2 and PSG5) to 8 cysteine residues (PSG10) which form from 2 (PSG2, 5, 11) to 3 disulphide bridges (see Table 1).

Table 1. Structural properties and functional modules of human pregnancy-specific glycoproteins.

Type of PSGs	Length, number of amino acid residues	Molecular weight, Da	Glycolysation sites	Disulphide bonds	Accession number in SwissProt/ TrEMBL data base
PSG1	419	47,223	N61, N104, N11, N199, N259,N268, N303	C169-C217, C262-C310, C354-C394	P11464
PSG2	335	37,216	N61, N104, N111, N199	C169-C217, C261-C301	P11465
PSG3	428	47,945	N104, N111, N199	C169-C217, C262-C310	Q16557
PSG4	419	47,045	N104, N111, N199, N268, N299, N303	C169-C217, C262-C310, C354-C394	Q6P520
PSG5	335	37,680	N104, N111, N175, N210	C169-C217, C261-C301	Q15238
PSG6	435	48,814	N61, N103, N110, N198, N267, N302, N381	C168-C216, C261-C309, C353-C393	Q00889
PSG7	419	47,001	N61, N104, N111, N199, N209, N268, N303	C169-C217, C262-C310, C354-C394	Q13046
PSG8	426	47,772	N61, N104, N111, N199, N268, N303	C169-C217, C262-C310, C354-C394	Q9UQ74
PSG9	426	48,272	N104, N111, N199, N268, N303, N387	C169-C217, C262-C310, C354-C394	Q00887
PSG10	424	47,501	N61, N103, N110, N198, N267, N302, N386, N419	C168-C216, C261-C309, C353-C419	Q15235
PSG11	332	36,881	N61, N104, N111	C169-C217, C261-C301	Q9UQ72

Searching through the GenBank and Swiss-Prot/TrEMBL databases revealed 74-80% homology between PSG1 cDNA and human carcinoembryonic antigen cDNA. PSG proteins have, similarly to CEACAMs, multi-domain structure. But the majority of PSGs lack membrane anchor and, therefore, are secreted into the blood [28]. Membrane-anchored CEACAMs are widely expressed during embryonic development and in adult tissues. They are implicated in multiple aspects of cell signalling, tissue homeostasis and disease, including carcinogenesis and regulation of immune and metabolic functions of the haemochorial placenta of rodents and primates [29].

Human as well as rodent PSGs are characterized by presence of several immunoglobulin(Ig)-like domains. With the exception of human PSG2 and PSG5, and mouse PSG24, PSG30, PSG31, structure all PSGs are based on a leader sequence and up to four Ig-like domains. These domains are designated: Ig-like V-type (or N), Ig-like C2-type 1 (or A1), Ig-like C2-type 2 (or A2) and Ig-like C2-type 3 (or B2) domain. The only type of domain found in all rodents and primates PSGs is the Ig-V(variable)-like domain located at amino terminus of polypeptide chain. This domain is also named N domain and shared by all members of the CEA family, suggesting that it contains important functional motifs [12].

Structure of the Ig-like domains of human and rodent PSGs differs [30]. Domain arrangements in human PSGs may be as follows: type I (N-A1-A2-B2-C), type IIa (N-A1-B2-C), type IIb (N-A2-B2-C), type III (N-B2-C) and type IV (A1-B2-C) [9]. Although human PSGs consist of only one N domain (Figure 1), rodents PSGs contain multiple such domains that are preceded by a short hydrophobic leader-like sequence [301]. For example, mouse PSGs are composed of 3 to 8 IgV-like N domains followed by one IgC-like A domain.

Pairwise comparison of all four domains of mouse PSGs with the all four domains of human PSGs indicates that amino acid residues of their N domains are the most conservative ones. The degree of homology between human and rodent N-terminal domains reaches 60%, which, as it has been shown, is sufficient for the ability of these proteins to induce cytokines. Notably, the homology within human PSGs is greater than 85%, which suggests that they might use the same receptor [32]. However, through binding to different receptors, human and murine PSGs may use identical signaling mechanisms that result in secretion of the same cytokines.

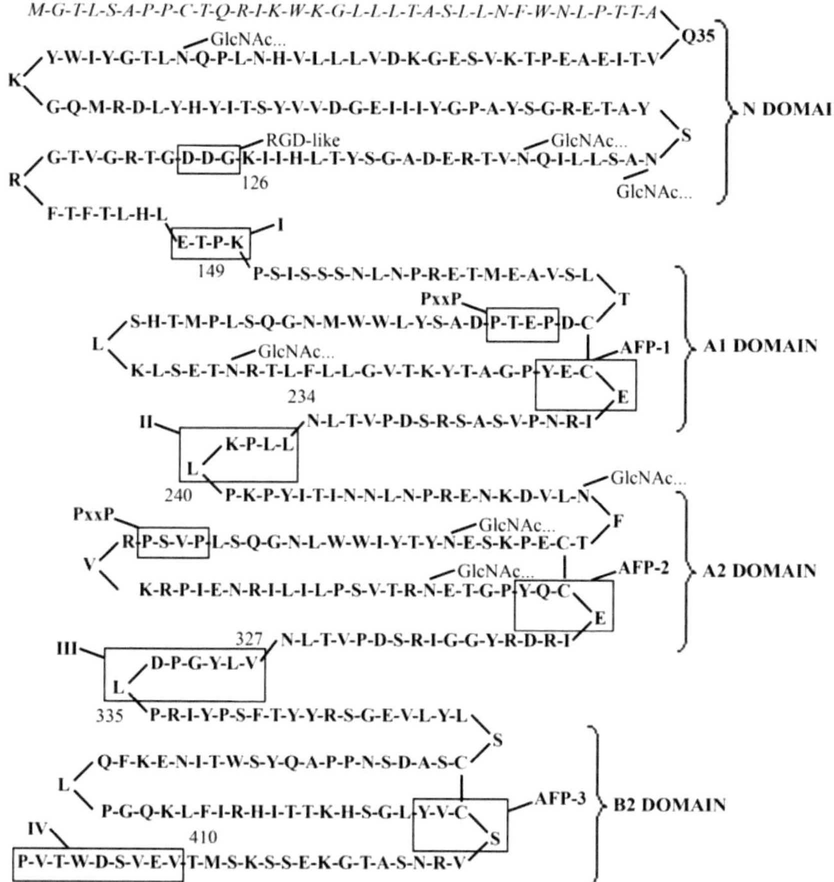

Signal peptide is shown *in italic* (amino acid residues 1-34). The tripeptide GGD (see text of the article) which corresponds to RGD is shown (amino acid (aa) residues 126-128). GlcNAc... is site of glycosylation (aa residues N61, N104, N111, N199, N259, N268, N303). I – first inter-domain peptide (aa residues 145-148), II – second inter-domain peptide (aa residues 235-239), III – third inter-domain peptide (aa residues 328-334), IV – C-terminal post-domain peptide (aa residues 411-419). PxxP motifs are also shown: in PGS1 these are sequences PETP, PKLP, PSVP and PDLP (amino acid residues 171-174, 281-284 and 332-335, respectively). The peptide PVSP is highly conserved and is present in all human PSGs. The two PxxP motifs are located in II and III inter-domain peptides. AFP-1, AFP-2, AFP-3 are AFP-like motifs (amino acid residues 215-218, 308-311, 392-395, respectively). There are also three disulphide bonds in PSG1 formed between C169-C217, C262-C310, and C354-C394.

Figure 1. Primary structure of human PSG1 with mapping of Ig-like domains and functional motifs.

Based on organization of N and A domains it has been proposed that the most probable PSG ancestor in rodents and primates is a CEACAM15-like molecule. CEACAM15 is not classified as a PSG because comparisons of N and A domain sequence identity clearly delineate members of the CEACAM and PSG subfamilies [33]. Relatively high conservation of primate N domains and rodent N1 domains confirms the fact that, despite independent gene family expansions and structural diversification, mouse and human PSGs retain conserved functions.

Biological/Physiological Functions of PSGs

The physiological functions of PSG proteins are not fully elucidated. Nevertheless, a number of experimental data and clinical observations allow supposing the critical role of PSGs in maintenance of pregnancy and their functional role during early embryo development and/or implantation. Currently, multiple lines of evidence suggest an immunomodulatory function for PSGs to prevent rejection of the allotypic fetus by maternal immune system. The immunoregulatory functions of PSG were first underscored by the observation that PSG suppresses the proliferative response of peripheral blood lymphocytes [34, 35]. Later it has been shown that human and mouse PSGs induce secretion of anti-inflammatory cytokines from monocytes and macrophages *in vitro* to regulate T cell activation and proliferation [36–38]. Treatment of monocytes with three members of human PSGs (PSG1, PSG6 and PSG11) induces secretion of interleukin (IL)-10, IL-6, and transforming growth factor-beta-1 (TGF-β1). The induction of anti-inflammatory cytokines by various PSGs supports the hypothesis that these glycoproteins have an essential role in regulation of the maternal immune response in biological species with hemochorial placentation [37].

It has been shown that recombinant isoform of PSG1 (PSG1a) being secreted to culture supernatants of infected HeLa cells is able to induce alternative activation of human peripheral blood monocytes. Recombinant PSG1a acts also as an important, accessory cell-dependent T cell suppressor factor inducing a partial growth arrest at the S/G2/M phase of cell cycle [38].

Also, PSG-mediated switching of immune system from a predominantly TH1 response to a predominantly TH2 response, which is considered more compatible with successful pregnancy, was observed [39]. It has been shown that mouse PSG18 is secreted from follicle-associated epithelium and is deposited in the subepithelium dome (SED) region. In addition, dendritic cells were found to highly express PSG receptor, namely CD9. The binding of mouse PSG to the CD9 has been reported to induce Th2 (IL-10 and IL-6) as well as Th3 (TGF-β1) cytokines in human monocytes and murine macrophages [40].

Likewise, recombinant Psg18 and its N-terminal domain (Psg18N) selectively unregulated IL-10 but not IL-1β, tumor necrosis factor (TNF)-α or IL-12p40 production in murine macrophages, even when co-stimulated with lipopolysaccharide, a potent inducer of proinflammatory cytokines [36].

There is extensive angiogenesis and vascular remodeling associated with pregnancy. Trophoblast giant cells produce a set of angiogenic, anti-angiogenic and vasoactive compounds. Some PSGs may exhibit angiogenic-related or vasoactivity functions. It has been shown that recombinant PSG23 induces TGF-β1, and vascular endothelial growth factor A (VEGF A) in primary murine macrophages and the macrophage cell line RAW 264.7. In addition, dendritic cells, endothelial cells, and trophoblasts, which are involved in maternal vasculature remodeling during pregnancy, secreted TGF-β1 and VEGF A in response to PSG23. Also, PSG23 showed cross-reactivity with human cells, including human monocytes and the trophoblast cell line, HTR-8/SVneo cells. So, PSGs can modulate the secretion of important pro-angiogenic factors, TGF-β1 and VEGF A, by different cell types involved in development of placenta [41].

Recently, it has been demonstrated that PSGs may play a role in reducing oxidative stress caused by toxic compounds in the blood to maintain cellular homeostasis during pregnancy. Over-expression of PSGs did not affect cell growth and morphology, but seemed to increase their resistance to a particular type of damaging agents. These agents capable of breaking single strand DNA associated with oxidative stress. It has been proposed that PSGs may exhibit coordinate expression during induced and replicative senescence [42].

Receptors for PSGs

The only PSGs receptor identified to date is the integrin-associated cluster of differentiation 9 antigen (CD9) receptor. In macrophages CD9 was found to bind the N1 domains of both PSG17 and PSG19 [43].The interaction of PSG17 and CD9 was found to be necessary for induction of secretion of anti-inflammatory cytokines. PSG17 has also been shown to prevent sperm–egg fusion by interrupting the binding of CD9 to a ligand on the egg surface [44]. Examination of temporal and spatial aspects of PSGs and CD9 expression during mouse pregnancy revealed that the PSGs and CD9 exhibited partial overlap in their expression, but without exlusive co-localization.

CD9 is widely expressed in the fetal compartments of the placenta and other uterine tissues throughout pregnancy. It has been shown that CD9 expression in pregnancy is not associated with immune cells, but, rather, with maternal decidual and vascular tissues [45]. This supports a scenario whereby PSGs secreted from fetal tissues interact with CD9 on maternal vasculature. However, whether this putative interaction would result in activation of signaling pathways relevant to endothelial cell function is unclear. An alternative scenario, based on the concept of maternal-fetal conflict [46], is that maternal CD9 expressed on vascular endothelium acts as a "sink" or decoy receptor for PSGs, thereby reducing the amount of PSGs available for interacting with maternal immune cells.

Human PSGs do not bind CD9, but nevertheless induce expression of a range of cytokines from monocytes similar to mouse PSGs [38]. The presence of the conserved tripeptide motif RGD (as described below) on a solvent-exposed loop in N-terminal Ig-like domain in the majority of human PSGs may indicate that this function involves integrin-related receptors [47]. It has also been speculated that the RGD-containing N-terminal domain may enable some PSGs for cell-matrix interactions [48]. Evidence supporting the hypothesis that the RGD-containing domain may be involved in receptor binding was provided by discovery that a peptide containing the RGD motif, from human PSG11, binds to a receptor on the surface of a promonocytic cell line [49]. By examining the U937 and THP-1 promonocyte cell lines, the presence of receptors with two different binding characteristics was demonstrated. The THP-1 receptor is identified by chemical cross-linking as a protein of 46 kilodaltons (kDa) and affinity chromatography demonstrates the presence of three protein species of 32 kDa, 16.8 kDa, and 15.9 kDa, suggesting the receptor has multiple subunits. In common with integrin interactions, this was dependent on the presence of bivalent cations and showed sensitivity to cytoskeletal signaling.

Binding to purified placental PSGs of normal human peripheral blood mononuclear cells activated with phorbol ester can be mimicked by a chemically synthesized peptide ligand. This peptide contains the RGD motif present at the N-terminal domain of PSG11. Receptors for PSG11 have been shown to be present on cells of the myeloid cell lineage, but not of T cell or B cell lineages [49]. The binding is mediated in part by RGD motif and can be competed by appropriate RGD-containing, but not RAD-containing, ligands.

Peptide Motifs and Biologically Active Sites

PxxP motif. It is recognized now that most proteins contain short linear peptide motifs which are associated with a particular function and are differed from globular protein domains [50]. A fraction of these linear amino acid sequences are, likely, linkers that provide correct spacing of domains in a protein. Many others are known to play pivotal functional roles. They may include sites for phosphorylation or glycosylation and other chemical modifications of proteins. Also, they may participate in protein-protein interactions including receptor-binding. An example is the canonical PxxP motif which is required for a protein binding to SH3 domains of signaling proteins such as protein kinases or adaptor proteins (c-Src and Grb2) [51−53]. In all human PSGs we found from 2 to 4 PxxP motifs (Table 2) in each protein. It may be speculated that the PxxP motifs facilitate signal transduction by PSG proteins through binding to adaptor proteins.

RGD and RGD-like motif. Most of human PSGs (except PSG1, PSG4 and PSG8) contain an integrin-binding tripeptide Arg-Gly-Asp (RGD) motif within their N-terminal domain that is thought to mediate interactions with the extracellular matrix and immune cells [54]. Human PSG1, PSG4, PSG8 contain RGD-like tripeptides, namely, GDD, RRD, GGD, correspondingly (Table 3). These RGD-like motifs are arisen by transition and transversion events during the evolution [12].

No rodent PSG isolated to date possesses an RGD domain. In contrast to the most human N domains, rodent N1 domains do not contain an RGD tri-peptide motif, but do contain RGD-like sequences. Rodent RGD-like motifs are represented by the following tripeptides in N1 domains: RCE, HCE and HAE, which are not conserved in rodent N2 and N3 domains. Such an an unexpected conservation of RGD-like motifs in N1 domain, which have been lost in N2 and N3 domains, may have functional significance.

$AFP_{14\text{-}20}$-like motifs. We found the following tetrapeptide motifs (YQCE, YECE, YACS) in almost all human PSGs which may also have functional importance (Table 3). One of these motifs (YQCE) is found in rodent (murine) PSGs. The consensus motif YxCx is a part of short heptapeptide LDSYQCT, which was found to be a biologically active site of human alpha-fetoprotein (AFP) [55]. The AFP-derived peptide fragment LDSYQCT ($AFP_{14\text{-}20}$) has been demonstrated to possess mmunomodulatory activity *in vitro*. Motifs similar to YxCx motif ($AFP_{14\text{-}20}$-like motifs) have also been found in growth factors of epidermal growth factor family (including EGF itself) and EGF-like modules of different cell adhesion molecules and coagulation factors [56].

Table 2. PxxP motifs in human pregnancy-specific glycoproteins.

Type of PSGs	PETP (aa residues)	PKLP (aa residues)	PVSP (aa residues)	PDLP (aa residues)
PSG1	171-174	237-240	281-284	332-335
PSG2	171-174	-	-	239-242
PSG3	171-174	237-240	281-284	332-335
PSG4	171-174 (PATP)	237-240 (PKLS)	281-284	332-335
PSG5	-	-	187-191	239-242
PSG6	170-173	236-239	280-283	331-334
PSG7	171-174	237-240	281-284	332-335
PSG8	171-174	237-240	281-284	332-335
PSG9	171-174 (PETL)	237-240	281-284	332-335
PSG10	170-173	236-239	280-283	331-334
PSG11	171-174	-	-	239-242

We studied the effect of PSG-derived peptides YACS (peptide A) and YACE (peptide Q) and CEA-derived peptide SYKCE on H1-histaminic and M-cholinic receptors in experimental model of ileum section contraction under the mediator influence. The peptide A suppressed reaction to both mediators on average of 10%. Peptide Q has considerable effect on average of 35% in suppression of contraction induced by histamine and stimulates reaction to acetylcholine on average of 20%. CEA-peptide, on the contrary, strengthened the contraction induced by histamine to 11% and suppressed acetylcholine effect by 16%. The double washing of ileum during 1–3 minutes completely abolished effects of the investigated peptides [57]. So, it may be concluded that both CEA- and PSG-derived peptides possess biological activity. The detailed physiological role of the tetrapeptide motifs (YQCE, YECE, YACS) found in all human PSGs is to be further elucidated.

Table 3. Putative functional motifs in human pregnancy-specific glycoproteins.

Type of PSGs	RGD (aa residues)	YECE (aa residues)	YQCE (aa residues)	YACS (aa residues)
PSG1	127-129 (GDD)	215-218	308-311	392-395 (YVCS)
PSG2	127-129	215-218	-	299-302 (YVCS)
PSG3	127-129	215-218	308-311	392-395
PSG4	127-129 (RRD)	215-218	308-311	392-395
PSG5	127-129	215-218	-	299-302 (YTCS)
PSG6	126-128	214-217	307-310	391-394
PSG7	127-129	215-218	308-311	392-395
PSG8	127-129 (GGD)	215-218	308-311	392-395
PSG9	127-129	215-218	308-311	392-395
PSG10	126-128	214-217	307-310	391-394
PSG11	127-129	215-218	-	299-302

Conclusion

Pregnancy-specific glycoproteins (PSGs) are secreted proteins which were first discovered as long as about 40 years ago. A number of experimental data and clinical observations together with correlation between low level of PSG and some defects in fetal development allow supposing their critical role in maintenance of pregnancy. However, structural and functional properties of PSGs have not been fully elucidated yet.

It has been shown that human as well as rodent PSGs may function as immunoregulatory proteins which regulate activity of T-lymphocytes and secretion of cytokines by monocytes and macrophages. Also, PGSs may cause maternal vasculature remodeling through influencing on secretion of pro-angiogenic agents such as transforming growth factor-beta1 (TGF-β1) and vascular endothelial growth factor (VEGF) by different cell types involved in the development of placenta.

Revealing of some peptide motifs in PSGs (such as RGD tripeptide, PxxP and AFP_{14-20}-like motifs) may indicate that they might play an important role in PSG functioning. They may provide binding to a receptor or other signaling proteins or may play a role of biologically active sites responsible for (at least in the part) immunomodulatory properties of PSGs.

References

[1] Rawn, S. M. & Cross, J. C. (2008). The evolution, regulation and function of placental-specific genes. *Rev. Cell Dev. Biol.*, *24*, 159-181.

[2] Cross, J. C., Baszyk, D., Dobric, N., Hemberger, M. & Hughes, M. (2003). Genes, development and evolution of the placenta. *Placenta*, *24*, 123-130.

[3] Rebstock S., Lucas K., Weiss M., Thompson J. & Zimmermann W. (1993). Spatiotemporal expression of pregnancy-specific glycoprotein gene rnCGM1 in rat placenta. *Dev. Dynamics*, *198*, 171-181.

[4] Kromer B., Finkenzeller, D., Wessels, J., Dveksler, G., Thompson, J. & Zimmermann, W. (1996). Coordinate expression of splice variants of the murine pregnancy-specific glycoprotein (PSG) gene family during placental development. *Eur. J. Biochem.*, *242*, 280-287.

[5] Lei, K. J., Sartwell, A. D., Pan, C. J. & Chou, J. Y. (1992). Cloning and expression of genes encoding human pregnancy-specific glycoproteins. *J. Biol. Chem.*, *267*, 16371-16378.

[6] Brummendorf, T. & Rathjen, F. G. (1994). Cell adhesion molecules. 1: immunoglobulin superfamily. *Prot. Profile*, *1*, 951-1058.

[7] Rudert, F., Zimmermann, W. & Thompson, J. A. (1989). Intra- and interspecies analyses of the carcinoembryonic antigen (CEA) gene family reveal independent evolution in primates and rodents. *J. Mol. Evol.*, *29*, 126-134.

[8] Teglund, S., Olsen, A., Khan, W. N., Frangsmyr, L. & Hammarstrom, S. (1994). The pregnancy-specific glycoprotein (PSG) gene cluster on human chromosome 19: fine structure of the 11 PSG genes and

identification of 6 new genes forming a third subgroup within the carcinoembryonic antigen (CEA) family. *Genomics*, *23*, 669-684.

[9] Teglund, S., Zhou, G. Q. & Hammarstrom, S. (1995). Characterization of cDNA encoding novel pregnancy-specific glycoprotein variants. *Biochem. Biophys. Res. Commun.*, *211*, 656-664.

[10] Thompson, J., Koumari, R., Wagner, K., Barnert, S., Schleussner, C., Schrewe, H., Zimmermann, W., Muller, G., Schempp, W. & Zaninetta, D. (1990). The human pregnancy-specific glycoprotein genes are tightly linked on the long arm of chromosome 19 and are coordinately expressed. *Biochem. Biophys. Res. Commun.*, *167*, 848-859.

[11] McLellan, A. S., Fischer, B., Dveksler, G., Hori, T., Wynne, F., Ball, M., Okumura, K., Moore, T. & Zimmermann, W. (2005). Structure and evolution of the mouse pregnancy-specific glycoprotein (Psg) gene locus. *BMC Genomics*, *6*, 4.

[12] McLellan, A. S., Zimmermann, W. & Moore, T. (2005). Conservation of pregnancy-specific glycoprotein (PSG) N-domains following independent expansions of the gene families in rodents and primates. *BMC Evol. Biol.*, *5*, 39.

[13] Zhou, G. Q., Baranov, V., Zimmermann, W., Grunert, F., Erhard, B., Mincheva-Nilsson, L., Hammarstrom, S. & Thompson, J. (1997). Highly specific monoclonal antibody demonstrates that pregnancyspecific glycoprotein (PSG) is limited to syncytiotrophoblast in human early and term placenta. *Placenta*, *18*, 491-501.

[14] Jurisicova, A., Antenos, M., Kapasi, K., Meriano, J. & Caper, R. F. (1999). Variability in the expression of trophectodermal markers beta-human chorionic gonadotrophin, human leucocyte antogen-G and pregnancy-specific beta 1- glycoprotein by the human blastocyst. *Hum. Reprod.*, *14*, 1852-1858.

[15] Avendano, C., Franchi, A., Jones, E. & Oehringer, S. (2009). Pregnancy-specific β1-glycoprotein 1 and human leucocyte antigen-E mRNA in human sperm: differential expression in ferile and infertile men and evidence of a possible functional role during early development. *Hum. Reprod.*, *24(2)*, 270-277.

[16] Chen, D. S., Asanaka, M., Yokomori, K., Wang, F., Hwang, S. B., Li, H. P. & Lai, M. M. (1995). A pregnancy-specific glycoprotein is expressed in the brain and serves as a receptor for mouse hepatitis virus. *Proc. Natl. Acad. Sci.*, USA, *92*, 12095-12099.

[17] Kawano, K., Ebisawa, M., Hase, M., Fukuda, S., Hujikata, A., Kawano, S., Date, Y., Tsuneda, S., Itoh, K. & Ohno, H. (2007). Psg18 is specifically expressed in follicle-associated epithelium. *Cell Struct. Funct., 32(2)*, 115-126.
[18] Tatarinov, Yu. S. & Masyukevich, V. N. (1970). Immunochemical identification of a new beta-1-globulin in the serum of pregnant women. *Bull.Exp. Biol. Med. (Rus.), 69(6)*, 66-68.
[19] Bohn, H. (1971). Detection and characterization of pregnancy proteins in the human placenta and their quantitative immunochemical determination in sera from pregnant women. *Arch. Gynakol., 210*, 440-457.
[20] Tatarinov, Yu. S., Mesnyankina, N. V., Nikulina, D. M., Novikova, L. A., Toloknov, B. O. & Falaleeva, D. M. (1974). Immunochemical identification of beta1-globulin of the "pregnancy zone" in serum of patients with trophoblastic tumors. *Int. J. Cancer, 14*, 548-554.
[21] Lin, T. M., Halbert, S. P. & Spellacy, W. N. (1974). Measurement of pregnancy-associated plasma proteins during human gestation. *J. Clin. Invest., 54*, 576-582.
[22] Hau, J., Gidley-Baird, A. A., Westergaard, J. G. & Teisner, B. (1985). The effect on pregnancy of intrauterine administration of antibodies against two pregnancy-associated murine proteins: murine pregnancy-specific 1-glycoprotein and murine pregnancy-associated 2-glycoprotein. *Biomed. Biochim. Acta, 44*, 1255-1259.
[23] Soares, M. J. (2004). The prolactin and growth hormone families: pregnancy-specific hormones/cytokines at the maternal-fetal interface. *Reprod. Biol. Endocrinol.*, **2**, 51.
[24] Silver, R. M., Heyborne, K. D. & Leslie, K. K. (1993) Pregnancy-specific β1-glycoprotein (SP-1) in maternal serum and amniotic fluid; pre-eclampsia, small for gestational age fetus and fetal distress. *Placenta, 14*, 583-589.
[25] Bohn, H. & Weinmann, E. (1976). [Antifertility effect of an active immunization of mokeys with human pregnancy-specific β1-glycoprotein (SP1)]. *Archiv. Gynakol., 221*, 305-312.
[26] Repina, M. A., Blagoslovenskii, G. S., Gnilevskaia, Z. U. & Ivanova, L. V. (1989). [The effect of specific trophoblastic beta 1-glycoprotein on changes in the cellular link of immunity in infected abortion]. *Akush. Ginekol., 12*, 47-50.

[27] Fialova, L., Kohoutova, B., Peliskova, Z., Malbohan, I. & Mikulikova, L. (1991). [Serum levels of trophoblast-specific beta-1-globulin (SP1) and alpha-1-fetoprotein (AFP) in pregnant women with rheumatoid arthritis]. *Cesk. Gynekol.*, *56*, 166-170.

[28] Han, E., Phan, D., Lo, P., Poy, M. N., Behringer, R., Najjar, S. M. & Lin, S. H. (2001). Differences in tissue-specific and embryonic expression of mouse Ceacam1 and Ceacam2 genes. *Biochem. J.*, *355*, 417-423.

[29] Zebhauser, R., Kammerer, R., Eisenried, A., McLellan, A., Moore, T. & Zimmermann, W. (2005). Identification of a novel group of evolutionary conserved members within the rapidly diverging murine CEA family. *Genomics*, *86*, 566-580.

[30] Thompson, J. A. (1995). Molecular cloning and expression of carcinoembryonic antigen gene family members. *Tumor Biol.*, *16*, 10-16.

[31] Zhou, G. Q. & Hammarstrom, S. (2001). Pregnancy-specific glycoprotein (PSG) in baboon (Papio hamadryas): family size, domain structure, and prediction of a functional region in primate PSGs. *Biol. Reprod.*, *64*, 90-99.

[32] Rooney, B. C., Horne, C. H. & Hardman, N. (1988). Molecular cloning of a cDNA for human pregnancy-specific β1-glycoprotein: homology with human carcinoembryonic antigen and related proteins. *Gene*, *71*, 439-449.

[33] Chan, W. Y., Bojigin, J., Zheng, Q. X. & Shupert, W. L. (1988). Characterization of cDNA encoding human pregnancy-specific beta 1-glycoprotein from placenta and extraplacental tissues and their comparison with carcinoembryonic antigen. *DNA*, *7*, 545-455.

[34] Majumdar, S., Bapna, B. C., Mapa, M. K., Gupta, A. N., Devi, P. K. & Subrahmanyam, D. (1982). Pregnancy-specific proteins: suppression of in vitro blastogenic response to mitogen by these proteins. *Internat.J. Fertil*, *27*, 66-69.

[35] Harris, S. J., Anthony, F. W., Jones, D. B. & Masson, G. M. (1984). Pregnancyspecific- beta 1-glycoprotein: effect on lymphocyte proliferation in vitro. *J. of Reprod. Immunol.*, *6*, 267-270.

[36] Wessells, J., Wessner, D., Parsells R., White, K., Finkenzeller, D., Zimmermann, W. & Dveksler, G. (2000). Pregnancy specific glycoprotein 18 induces IL-10 expression in murine macrophages. *Eur. J. Immunol.*, *30*, 1830-1840.

[37] Snyder, S. K., Wessner, D. H., Wessells, J. L., Waterhouse, R. M., Wahl, L. M., Zimmermann, W. & Dveksler, G. S. (2001). Pregnancy-specific glycoproteins function as immunomodulators by inducing secretion of IL-10, IL-6 and TGF-beta1 by human monocytes. *Am. J. Reprod. Immunol.*, *45*, 205-216.

[38] Motran, C. C., Diaz, F. L., Gruppi, A., Slavin, D., Chatton, B. & Bocco, J. L. (2002). Human pregnancy-specific glycoprotein 1a (PSG1a) induces alternative activation in human and mouse monocytes and suppresses the accessory cell-dependent T cell proliferation. *J. Leukoc. Biol.*, *72*, 512-521.

[39] Motran, C. C., Diaz, F. L., Montes, C. L., Bocco, J. L. & Gruppi, A. (2003). In vivo expression of recombinant pregnancy-specific glycoprotein 1a induces alternative activation of monocytes and enhances Th2-type immune response. *Eur. J. Immunol.*, *33*, 3007-3016.

[40] Ha, C. T., Waterhouse, R., Wessells, J., Wu, J. A. & Dveksler, G. S. (2005). Binding of pregnancy-specific glycoprotein 17 to CD9 on macrophages induces secretion of IL-10, IL-6, PGE2, and TGF-beta1. *J. Leukoc. Biol.*, *77*, 948-957.

[41] Wu, J. A., Johnson, B. L., Chen, Y., Ha, C. T. & Dveksler, G. S. (2008). Murine pregnancy-specific glycoprotein 23 induces the proangiogenic factors transforming growth factor beta 1 and vascular endothelial growth factor in a cell types involved in vascular remodeling in pregnancy. *Biol. Reprod.*, *79(6)*, 1054-1061.

[42] Endoh, M., Kobayashi, Y., Yamakami, Y., Yonekura, R., Fujii, M. & Ayusawa, D. (2009). Coordinate expression of the human pregnancy-specific glycoprotein gene family during induced and replicative senescence. *Biogerontology*, *10(2)*, 213-221.

[43] Waterhouse, R., Ha, C. & Dveksler, G. S. (2002). Murine CD9 is the receptor for pregnancy-specific glycoprotein 17. *J. Exp. Med.*, *195*, 277-282.

[44] Ellerman, D. A., Ha, C., Primakoff, P., Myles, D. G. & Dveksler, G. S. (2003). Direct binding of the ligand PSG17 to CD9 requires a CD9 site essential for sperm-egg fusion. *Mol. Biol. Cell*, *14*, 5098-5103.

[45] Wynne, F., Ball, M., McLellan, A. S., Dockery, P., Zimmermann, W. & Moore, T. (2006). Mouse pregnancy-specific glycoproteins: tissue-specific expression and evidence of association with maternal vasculature. *Reproduction*, *131*, 721-732.

[46] Haig, D. (1993). Genetic conflicts in human pregnancy. *Quater. Rev. Biol.*, *68*, 495-532.

[47] McLenachan, P. A., Lockhart, P. J., Faber, H. R. & Mansfield, B. C. (1996). Evolutionary analysis of the multigene pregnancy-specific beta 1-glycoprotein family: separation of historical and nonhistorical signals. *J. Mol. Evol.*, *42*, 273-280.

[48] Khan, W. N., Teglund, S., Bremer, K. & Hammarstrom, S. (1992). The pregnancyspecific glycoprotein family of the immunoglobulin superfamily: identification of new members and estimation of family size. *Genomics*, *12*, 780-787.

[49] Rutherfurd, K. J., Chou, J. Y. & Mansfield, B. C. (1995). A motif in PSG11s mediates binding to a receptor on the surface of the promonocyte cell line THP-1. *Mol. Endocrinol.*, *9*, 1297-1305.

[50] Neduva, V. & Russell, R.B. (2005) Linear motifs: evolutionary interaction switches. *FEBS Lett. 579*, 3342-3345.

[51] Mayer, B. (2001). SH3 domains: complexity in moderation. *J. Cell Sci.*, *114(7)*, 1253-1263.

[52] Ghose, R., Shektman, A., Goger, M. J., Ji, H. & Cowburn, D. (2001). A novel, specific interaction involving the Csk SH3 domain and its natural ligand. *Nat. Struct. Biol.*, *8*, 998-1004.

[53] Solomaha, E., Szeto, F. L., Youself, M. A. & Palfrey, H. C. (2005). Kinetics of Src homology 3 domain association with the proline-rich domain of dynamins: specificity, occlusion, and the effects of phosphorylation. *J. Biol. Chem.*, *280*, 23147-23156.

[54] Ruoslahti, E. & Peirsbacher, M. D. (1987). New perspectives in cell adhesion: RGD and integrins. *Science*, *238*, 491-497.

[55] Terentiev, A. A. & Moldogazieva, N. T. (2006). Structural and functional mapping of alpha-fetoprotein. *Biochemistry (Mosc.)*, *71(2)*, 120-132.

[56] Terentiev, A. A. & Moldogazieva, N. T. (2007). Cell Adhesion Proteins and alpha-Fetoprotein. Similar Structural Motifs as Prerequisites for Common Functions. *Biochemistry (Mosc.)*, *72(9)*, 920-935.

[57] Terentiev, A. A., Moldogazieva, N. T., Tagirova, A. K. & Kazimirsky, A. N. (2008). Biological Activity and Dynamic Properties of Human Alpha-Fetoprotein-Derived Peptide LDSYQCT. *Tumor Biol.*, *29, S.1*, 74.

In: Human Placenta: Structure and Development... ISBN: 978-1-60876-457-0
Editors: E. Berven, et al. pp. 145-159 © 2010 Nova Science Publishers, Inc.

Chapter V

Regulatory Action of Protein Inhibitors from Tubers of Potato Solanum Tuberosum L. to Transpeptidase Activity of Fibrin Stabilizing Factor (FXIIIa)

E.A. Kostanova*[*]*, M.A. Rozenfel'd and S.D. Varfolomeev
Institute of Biochemical Physics of the Russian Academy of Sciences, 119991, Moscow, 4 Kosygin St.

Abstract

Thrombosis and thromboembolism of various etiology, which are conditioned by activation of blood clotting factors and of fibrin stabilizing factor (FXIIIa) especially, are among the most severe and widespread kinds of blood-clotting pathologies. The last one catalyzes formation of γ-glutamyl-ε-lysin cross link reactions at the sites of α- and γ-polypeptide chains of fibrin molecules. For there are no physiologic inhibitors of FXIIIa, uncontrolled elevation of its enzymatic activity leads to hyper stability of thrombus to plasmin hydrolysis and makes fibrinolytic therapy ineffective. This fact determines importance to search ways of FXIIIa transpeptidase activity regulation using various

[*] Corresponding author: e-mail: ibcp@sky.chph.ras.ru, kostanova51@mail.ru

approaches from outside. The ability of cysteine proteinase inhibitors (CPIs) isolated from tubers of potato (Solanum tuberosum L.) to suppress transpeptidase activity of fibrin stabilizing factor (FXIIIa) through the direct effect on the essential SH group of the enzyme active site has been studied. The formation of fibrin clots soluble in 5 M urea and 2% acetic acid as well as spectrophotometric turbidity analysis of the stabilization and resistance of fibrin clots formed in the presence of FXIIIa and CPIs from potato tubers to plasmin, and electrophoresis of reduced fibrin and casein samples indicate the decrease or absence of covalent cross-linking of fibrin and casein chains. In addition, CPIs added to the substrate proved to decelerate fibrinogen polymerization almost twice relative to control. It is concluded that natural CPIs can both take part in the regulation of FXIIIa transpeptidase activity *in vitro* and modify the substrate.

Keywords: Cystein proteinase inhibitors (CPIs), fibrin stabilizing factor (FXIII), transpeptidase activity.

Introduction

To date, factor XIII (FXIII, fibrin stabilizing factor or fibrinoligase) is the best studied transglutaminase, and its physiological role has been determined [1]. Factor XIII is a plasma protein circulating as an a_2b_2 tetramer with a molecular weight of 320 kDa; two *a* subunits are catalytically active, while two *b* subunits are not. The molecular weight of the subunits is similar (about 80 kDa). The *b* subunits in FXIII were shown to stabilize the *a* subunits [2,3].

In contrast to many transglutaminases, FXIII is a proenzyme that becames active after proteolytic attack of thrombin in the presence of fibrin [4]. The active enzyme (a_2' or FXIIIa) is accumulated at the final stage of the blood clotting cascade through the cleavage of the activation peptide (4000 Da) from the N-terminus of each *a* subunit [2, 5]. In the presence of Ca^{2+}, the $a_2'b_2$ tetramer dissociates into the active dimmer (a_2') and two *b* subunits [3, 6, 7]. Calcium ions bind to the a' subunits and thus expose the active regions in the enzyme molecule [6, 8].

FXIIIa contains a cysteine in the active site; however, in contrast to thiol proteinases such as papain or catepsins B, H and L that hydrolyze peptide bonds, this transpeptidase forms intramolecular γ-glutamyl-ε-lysine crosslinks between fibrin molecules, which mechanically stabilize the fibrin clot and make it resistant to proteolysis [9].

Insoluble fibrin production directly depends on FXIIIa activity. For instance, low enzyme activity results in the formation of defective clots that readily dissolve in 5 M urea or 2% acetic acid, which can cause bleeding [10]. This process underlies bleeding in congenial or acquired FXIII deficiency. As FXIIIa activity increases, it is involved in pathological processes such as atherosclerosis, tumor growth, metastasis, respiratory distress syndrome in newborn babies, and other thrombotic disorders [11, 12].

As soon as FXIIIa is produced at the final stage of the coagulation cascade, various inducers and inhibitors can modulate its regulatory activity . To date, little is known about the nature of such factors in biological environment; however, *in vitro* experiments can shed light on some of their properties.

According to current views, transglutaminase activity of FXIII can be regulated at the enzyme level and at the substrate level, and this regulation has different forms [13]. The main structural requirements for inhibitors of fibrinogen cross-linking were formulated by Nilsson et al. [14]. A number of inhibitors highly specific for the cross-linking enzyme were specified [15, 13]. The basic idea of selecting FXIII inhibitors is that any specific inhibitor can bind to the cysteine in the active site before crosslinking reaction. However, all known compounds used to inhibit FXIII cross-linking activity with direct effect on the enzyme active site are not natural.

Natural protein inhibitors of proteinases are widespread in the plant and animal world. They represent a special group of proteins sharing the capacity to form protein-protein complexes, which competitively inhibits the catalytic activity. Protein inhibitors have been identified in food, particularly, seeds of legumes, cereals, and olive family as well as fruits, vegetables, potatoes, milk, and various animal tissues. The properties and functions of most of them are well known [16, 17]. Proteinase inhibitors were long considered as anti-dietary factors; however, they have recently become interesting for their possible anticancer [18] and positive dietary effects [19]. In particular, antipain proved to inhibit carcinogen-induced malignant transformation *in vitro* [20-23], while proteinase inhibitors from potato act as anticancer agents affecting tumor cell growth (proliferation) [23], H_2O_2 production [24], and processes induced by solar UV radiation [25].

In tubers of potato (*Solanum tuberosum L.*), proteinase inhibitors amount to 30% of total protein [26]. In addition to inhibitors of serine and aspartate proteinases as well as carboxypeptidase inhibitor, potato tubers contain considerable quantities of cysteine proteinase inhibitors. These inhibit papain, lysosomal cathepsins B, H, and L through the interaction with these enzymes in equimolar amounts [27, 28].

Considering that FXIII is a thiol enzyme similar to papain in many respects, the goal of this work was to study the ability of protein inhibitors of cystein proteinases from potato tubers to modulate transpeptidase activity of the enzyme *in vitro.*

Materials and Methods

Fibrinogen was isolated from citrate bovine plasma and purified from plasminogen and fibrin stabilizing factor as described elsewhere [29].

Fibrin stabilizing factor was isolated from bovin blood as described by Lorand et al. [30]. Its activity determined by the method of Loewy and Dunathan [31] was 320 U/ml (1 U corresponds to FXIIIa activity in 1 ml donor serum). FXIII was converted to active FXIIIa by the addition of 15 NIH/ml thrombin (Roche, France) to a final concentration of 7.5 NIH/ml; the mixture was incubated at 25°C for 10 min.

Plasminogen was isolated from human plasma by affinity chromatography on lysine Sepharose 4B (Pharmacia, Sweden) [32].

Plasmin was obtained by plasminogen activation by streptase (Behringwerke, Germany) as described previously [33]. The sample activity was determined by casein digestion assay [34]; it equaled 12 casein U/mg protein.

Whole casein was prepared as described by Lavies and Low [35] from skim-milk of cows.

The inhibitors were isolated from tubers of potato cultivar Istrinskii harvested in 2003. The tubers were processed as described elsewhere [27] and the protein fraction after centrifugation was applied to an affinity chromatography column. KM-chymopapain was used as the affinity sorbent to isolate CPIs for the first time. It was synthesized using the standart technique [36]. Multiple forms of chymopapain were isolated from the water-soluble latex fraction from crude fruits of papaya (*Carica papaya)* as described previously [37, 38]. Proteolytic activity of immobilized chymopapain was determined in a thermostatted cell at 37°C with continious stirring. Casein supplemented with Lcysteine and ethylendiaminetetraacetic acid (EDTA) was used as substrate. Proteolytic activity assay of immobilized chymopapain demonstrated that the active enzyme concentration was 0.6-0.8 mg/ml Sepharose. The activity of the isolated inhibitors was determined in mixtures containing constant quantities of chymopapain, papain (Merck, Germany), or ficin (Calbiochem, US) and different inhibitor quantities (total volume of 1 ml) incubated at 37°C for 10 min in 0.5 M Tris-HCI, pH 8.0 with 0.005 M L-cysteine and 0.002 M EDTA, after which 1 ml of substrate was added. The residual proteolytic activity of thiol enzymes used as control was determined by the modified Kunitz method [39]. Electrophoresis in 20% polyacrylamide gel with 1% sodium dodecyl sulphate (SDS) and 1% 2-mercaptoethanol was performed according to Laemmli [40]. Lactoglobulin, soybean Kunitz inhibitor, carbonic anhydrase, ovalbumin, bovin serum albumin, and phosphorylase B (Serva, Germany) were used as molecular weight markers.

The effect of CPIs on the physicochemical properties of fibrin clot in the presence of FXIIIa was studied by monitoring the turbidity during the clotting period.

The polymerization rate was turbidimetrically measured as follows: 3.0 ml of 0.09 mg/ml fibrinogen in 0.05 M Tris, pH 7.4, 0.15 M NaCI, and 5mM $CaCI_2$ was supplemented with 0.075 ml thrombin with the activity of 15 NIH/ml.

The rate of fibrinogen stabilization was turbidimetrically determined after the addition of 0.01 ml FXIIIa (160 U/ml) and CPIs from potato tubers to the abovementioned reaction mixture at 1 : 0, 1 : 0.5, 1 : 1, and 1 : 1.5 (w/w). In both cases, the mixtures were immediately agitated and the absorption changes at 350 nm were monitored on a UV VIS Specord (Carl Zeiss Jena, Germany). The solubility of the resulting fibrin clots in 5 M urea and 2% acetic acid [31, 41] was estimated visually.

The resistance to plasmin of fibrin clots, to a different extent polymerized by FXIIIa, inhibited by CPIs from potato tubers was also determined turbidimetrically after the addition of 0.075 ml plasmin (0.9 casein U) to the reaction mixture.

Fibrin and casein chains were covalently cross-linked by the addition of 0.01 ml of activated FXIIIa (1.6 U/ml) or FXIIIa to a different extent inactivated by CPIs (at 1 : 0, 1 : 0.5, 1 :1, and 1 : 1.5 w/w), and 0.075 ml of thrombin for fibrin to 0.6 ml and to 0.05 ml each kind of substrate respectively. The cross-linking reaction was performed in 0.05 M Tris, pH 7.4, 0.15 M NaCI, and 5 mM $CaCI_2$ for 15 min at 37°C. The fibrin cross-linking reaction was stopped by a mixture of 8 M urea, 2% SDS, and 5% 2-mercaptoethanol and the casein cross-linking reaction was stopped. with the same mixture without adding urea. The degree of chain cross-linking of fibrin and casein was estimated by SDS electrophoresis of the reduced samples in 7.5% [42] and 12.5 % [40] polyacrylamide gels, respectively.

Protein was quantified by the modified Bradford method [43].

Results and Discussion

The electrophoretic profiles of protein inhibitors isolated from potato tubers by affinity chromatography on CM-chymopapain Sepharose 4B (Figure 1) demonstrate that CPIs include many protein forms of different molecular weight and quantities. The inhibition of thiol proteinases (papain, chymopapain, and ficin) by increasing CPI quantities is shown in Figure 2. The activity was completely blocked at the inhibitor-enzyme ratio of 1 : 1 for chymopapain and ficin and of 1 : 2 for papain (w/w). Thus, the inhibitors isolated from potato tubers are proteins with a high specificity for thiol proteinases.

The turbidity monitoring during the clotting period allowed us to indirectly identify different stages in fibrin polymerization and stabilization *in vitro* in the presence of CPIs from potato tubers. Figure 3 demonstrates that the addition of the inhibitors to the reaction mixture containing fibrinogen, thrombin, and Ca^{2+} ions decreased the rate of turbidity changes more than twice and reduced the lag period nearly twice as well (Figure 3, curve *3*) compared to control (Figure 3, curve 1). The addition of FXIIIa inhibited by CPIs from potato tubers to the reaction mixture containing fibrinogen, thrombin, and Ca^{2+} demonstrates that the deceleration of the turbidity changes (Figure 3, curve *2*) depended on the inhibitor quantities. This result allows us to propose that CPIs inhibit the enzyme activity of FXIIIa. In order to confirm this proposal, the degree of stabilization of fibrin clots formed by reactions shown in Figure 3 was evaluated by their solubility in 5 M urea and 2% acetic acid [31, 41]. Visual inspection demonstrated that stabilized fibrin clot was resistant to enzyme hydrolysis in the presence of plasmin (Figure 3, curve *2*). At the same time, unsubsidized fibrin formed in the presence of the maximum inhibitor concentration readily dissolved in the above-mentioned solvents (Figure 3, curves *1, 3, 6*). Stabilized fibrin formed in the presence of CPIs at 1

: 0.5 and 1 : 1 enzyme-inhibitor ratios (w/w) was partially soluble (Figure 3, curves *4,5*).

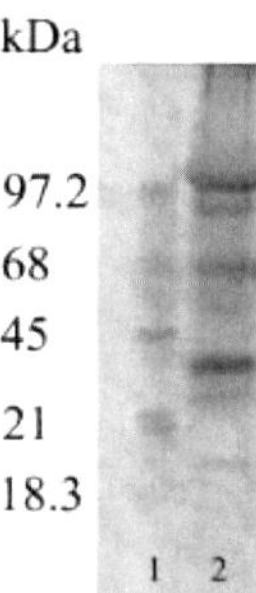

Figure 1. Electrophoresis of reduced samples of CPIs isolated from potato tubers by affinity chromatography on CM-chymopapain Sepharose 4B: *1*- protein markers, *2*- CPIs.

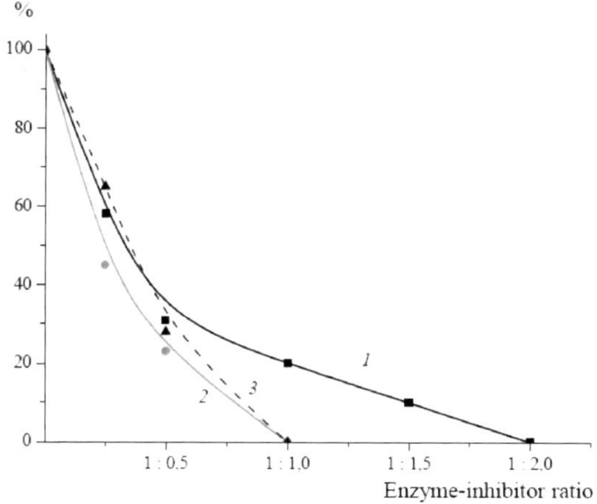

Figure 2. Effect of CPIs on the activity of: *1* – papain, *2* – ficin, *3* – chymopapain; casein was used as a substrate in enzyme activity assay; ordinate – residual proteolytic activity, %.

Figure 4 demonstrates the kinetic measurements of enzyme hydrolysis of fibrin clots cross-linked by FXIIIa to a different extent inhibited by CPIs from potato tubers. The clots formed in the presence of FXIIIa and CPIs at 1 : 0.5 and 1 : 1 ratios are lysed by plasmin after 30 and 25 min, respectively; while the clot stabilized by FXIIIa in the absence of the inhibitors is resistant to enzyme hydrolysis.

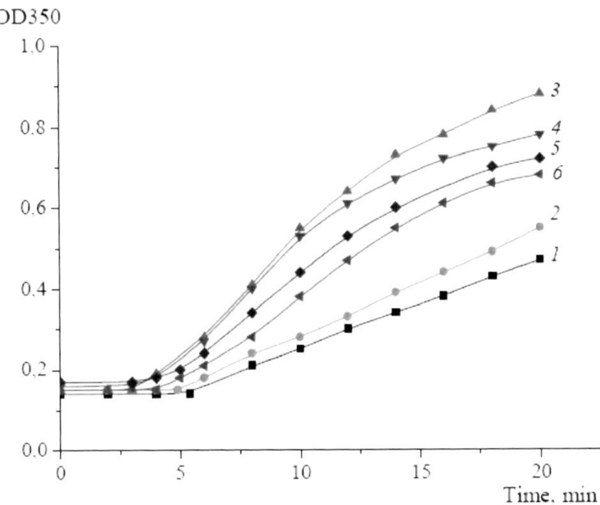

Figure 3. Monitoring fibrin clot turbidity. Optical dencity (OD) at 350 nm in time (min) in the presence of: *1* - thrombin, *2* – thrombin and FXIIIa, *3* – thrombin and CPIs; *4, 5, 6*, - thrombin, FXIIIa, and CPIs at enzyme - inhibitor ratios of 1 : 0.5, 1 : 1, and 1 : 1.5 (w/w), respectively.

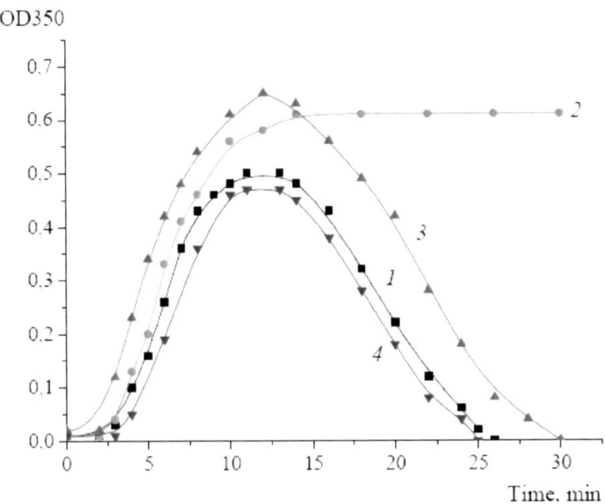

Figure 4. Turbidity monitoring during clot hydrolysis by plasminogen. Optical density (OD) at 350 nm in time (min) in the presence of: *1*- thrombin, *2* – thrombin and FXIIIa, *3, 4* – thrombin and FXIIIa inhibited by CPIs at enzyme - inhibitor ratios of 1 : 0.5 and 1 : 1 (w/w), respectively.

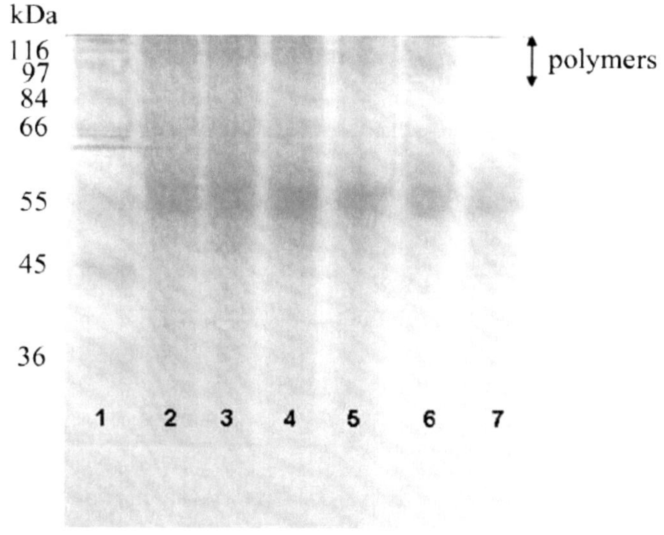

Figure 5. Electrophoresis of reduced samples of reaction product of casein crosslinking by FXIIIa with CPIs absence and in conditions of their presence in various concentrations: 1 – protein markers, 2 –wall casein, 3 – casein and FXIIIa, 4,5,6,7 – casein and FXIIIa inhibited by CPIs at enzyme-inhibitor ratios of 1 : 03, 1 : 07, 1 : 1 and 1 : 1,5 (w/w) respectively.

Casein was used as a nonspecific substrate in order to show CPIs isolated from tubers of potato impact exactly the direct effect on the essential SH-group of the enzyme active site of FXIIIa. It had been recently established by many researchers that particularly β-casein and some of its derivates, which in their amino-acid structure contain glutamine residuals, appear an excellent substrate for FXIIIa [48-51].

Figure 5 shows under FXIIIa influence which is inhibited by CPIs in various rates, retardation of covalent process of casein polypeptide chains' ligation, while polymer synthesis decreases or is absolutely absent on the enzyme-inhibitor weight relation in 1 : 0, 1 : 0.3, 1: 0,7, 1 : 1 and 1: 1,5.

This is also confirmed by electrophoretic profile of the reduced samples of chains (Figure 6). A decelerated involvement of the γ- and α-chains in crosslinking mediated by FXIIIa to a different extent inhibited by CPIs from potato tubers was observed, while the proportion of hybrid α-γ-chains and α-polymers was low or zero in stabilized fibrin.

It is common knowledge that fibrinogen molecule is a dimmer composed of three pairs of protein chains (*Aα, Bβ, and* γ_2) that form five main domains:

the central domain (*E*), two peripheral domains (*D*), and two αC domains. The main function of fibrinogen is formation of insoluble fibrin, which occurs in several stages. First, thrombin cleaves two pairs of fibrinopeptides *A* and *B* from the fibrinogen molecule, which opens polymerization sites in the central domain *E*. The complementary centers are localized in the domains *D* and require no enzyme activation. Spontaneous polymerization of fibrin monomers results in spatially regular linear two-stranded protofibrils, where each *D* domain of one molecule laterally associates with the central domain *E* of the second molecule and end-to-end contacts the *D* domain of the third one, thus, forming a "tridomain" node *D-E-D*. At the final stages of self-assembly, protofibrils aggregate to form ramified fibrils [44, 45], which forms the basis of the three-dimensional fibrin gel. The addition of protein inhibitors from potato tubers to fibrinogen in the presence of thrombin and Ca^{2+} decelerated polymerization of monomeric fibrin. Clearly, these protein inhibitors can interact with fibrinogen molecules and monomeric fibrin and induce local conformational transformations of the substrate molecules, thus, indirectly affecting the polymerization sites.

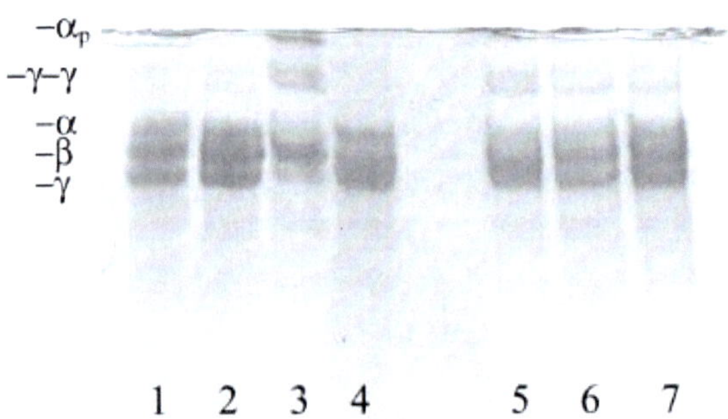

Figure 6. Electrophoresis of reduced samples of unstabilized (*1, 2, 4*) and stabilized (*3, 5, 6, 7*) fibrin in the presence of 1–fibrinogen; 2- thrombin; 3 – thrombin and FXIIIa; 4 – thrombin and CPIs; 5, 6, 7 – thrombin and FXIIIa ihibited by CPIs at enzyme – inhibitor ratios of 1 : 0.5, 1 : 1, and 1 : 1.5 (w/w), respectively.

Activated fibrin stabilizing factor crosslinks the γ- and α-chains of monomeric fibrin through the formation of ε/γ-glutamyl-lysine covalent bonds. In this case, the C-terminal regions of the γ-chains in mutually contacting *D* domains are responsible for the generation of intramolecular γ-dimers, while α- chains of monomeric fibrin associate with α-chains of two more molecules, which results in α-polymers [46, 47]. The $\beta\beta$-chains are not involved in cross linking. FXIIIa to a different extent inhibited by CPIs from potato tubers decelerates the involvement of γ- and α-chains in fibrin covalent cross-linking. In this case, intermolecular γ-dimers are formed in the stabilized fibrin molecule, while the proportion of α-polymers and hybrid α-γ-chains is low or zero at the enzyme – inhibitor ratio of 1 : 1.5 (w/w).

The solubility in 5 M urea and 2% acetic acid and low resistance of fibrin clots to hydrolysis by plasmin coupled with the data on the inhibition of ε/γ-glutamyl-lysine covalent bonds unambiguously confirm the ability of these protein inhibitors to suppress transpeptidase activity of the enzyme.

The obtained data suggest that CPIs from potato *S. tuberosum* tubers are physiologically active natural compounds that can specifically regulate activities of the endogenous and exogenous proteinases including FXIIIa. These protein inhibitors were shown to inhibit in one step both proteolytic activity of cysteine proteinases (papain, chymopapain, and ficin) and transpeptidase activity of FXIIIa *in vitro*.

Thus, we have isolated the total fraction of protein inhibitors of cysteine proteinases from potato tubers using CM-chymopapain Sepharose 4B and used them to study the regulation of FXIIIa transpeptidase activity *in vitro*. These protein inhibitors proved both to modify the substrate, apparently, through the impact on the polymerization sites of monomeric fibrin, and to inhibit crosslinking of α- and γ-chains of fibrin through the direct impact on the FXIIIa active site.

Regulation of the enzymatic activity of FXIIIa by inhibitors of natural origin, which are possess with a direct effect on the enzyme active site, presents the significant problem as well as in fundamental and practical medicine, particularly, the future investigations in this area can be assist the creation of therapeutic facilities have an influence on thrombogenesis process.

References

[1] Ichinose, A., Bottenus, R. E. & Davic, E. W. (1990). Structure of Transglutaminases. *J.Biol.Chem.*, *265(23)*, 13411-113414.

[2] Schwartz, M. L., Pizzo, S. V., Hill, R. L. & Mc Kee, P. A. (1973). The subunit structures of human plasma and platelet Factor XIII (Fibrinstabilizing Factor). *J.Biol. Chem.*, *248*, 1395-1407.

[3] Chung, S. I., Lewis, M. S. & Folk, J. E. (1974). Relationships of the catalytic properties of human plasma and platelet transglutaminases (activated blood coagulation Factor XIII) to their subunit structure. *J. Biol. Chem.*, *249*, 940-950.

[4] Lewis, S. D., Janus, T. J., Lorand, L. & Shafer, J. A. (1985). Regulation of formation of Factor XIIIa by its fibrin substrates. *Biochemistry*, *24*, 6772-6777.

[5] Takagi, T. & Doolittle, R. F. (1974). Aminoacid sequence studies of plasmin-derived fragments of human fibrinogen: amino-terminal sequences of intermediate and terminal fragments. *Biochemistry*, *13*, 750-756.

[6] Cooke, R. D. (1974). Calcium-induced dissociation of human plasma Factor XIII and the appearance of catalytic activity. *Biochem. J.*, *141*, 683-691.

[7] Lorand, L., Gray, A. J., Brown, K., et al., (1974). Dissociation of the subunit structures of fibrin stabilizing factor during activation of the zymogen. *Biochem. Biophys. Res. Commun.*, *56*, 914-922.

[8] Curtis, C. G., Brown, K. L., Credo, R. B., et al., (1974). Calcium dependent unmasking of active centre cysteine during activation of fibrin stabilizing factor. *Biochemistry*, *13*, 3774-3780.

[9] Takahashi, N., Takahashi, Y. & Putnam, F. W. (1986). Primary structure of blood coagulation Factor XIIIa (fibrinoligase, transglutaminase) from human placenta. *Proc. Natl. Acad. Sci.*, USA, *83*, 8019-8023.

[10] Nussbaum, M. & Morse, B., (1964). Plasma fibrin stabilizing factor activity in various diseases. *Blood*, *23*, 669-675.

[11] Muzbek, L. & Laki, K. (1984). Interaction of thrombin with proteins other than fibrinogen (thrombin, susceptible bonds). Activation of Factor XIII. In *Thrombin*, R. Machovich, Ed., Boca Raton EL: CRC Press, 83-102.

[12] McDonagh, J. (1982). Structure and function of Factor XIII. In *Hemostasis and Trombosis: Basic Principles and Clinical Practic,* R. W. Colman, J. Hirsh, V. J. Marder, et al., (Eds.), Philadelphia: Lippincott, 164-173.

[13] Lorand, L. & Conrad, S. M. (1984). Transglutaminases. *Mol. Cell. Biochem.*, *58*, 9-35.

[14] Nilsson, J. L. G., Stenberg, P., Ljunggren, C. & Hofman, R. J. (1972). *Ann. New York Acad. Sci.*, *202*, 286-296.

[15] Lorand, L., Rule, N. G., Ong, H. H., et al., (1968). Amine specificity in transpeptidation. Inhibition of fibrin cross-linking. *Biochemistry*, *7*, 1214-1223.

[16] Mosolov, V. V. & Valueva, T. A. (1993). *Rastitel'nye belkovye ingibitory proteoliticheskikh fermentov* (Plant protein inhibitors of proteolytic enzymes), Moscow: INBI.

[17] Valueva, T. A. & Mosolov, V. V. (2002). The role of proteolytic enzyme inhibitors in plant defense. *Usp. Biol. Khim.(Russia)*, *42*, 193-216.

[18] Kennedy, A. R. (1998). Chemopreventive agents: Protease inhibitors. *Pharmocol. Ther.*, *78(3)*, 167-209.

[19] Hill, A. J., Peikin, S. R., Ryan, C. A. & Dong, Z. G. (1990). Oral administration of protease Inhibitor II from potatoes reduces energy intake in man. *Physiol. Behav.*, *48*, 241-246.

[20] Borek, C., Miller, R. C., Pain, C. & Troll, W. (1979). Conditions for inhibiting and enhancing effects of the protease inhibitor antipain on Xray-induced neoplastic transformation in hamster and mouse cells. *Proc. Natl. Acad. Sci.*, USA, *76*, 6699-6707.

[21] Di Paolo, J. A., Amsbaugh, S. C. & Popescu, N. C. (1980). Antipain inhibits N- methyl-N′-nitrosoguanidine-induced transformation and increases chromosomal aberrations. *Proc. Natl. Acad. Sci.*, USA, *77*, 6649-6653.

[22] Kuroki, T. & Dreven, C. (1979). Inhibition of chemical transformation of C3H/10T1/2 cells by protease inhibitors. *Cancer. Res.*, *39*, 2755-2761.

[23] Blanco-Aparicio, C., Molina, M. A., Fernandez-Salas, E., et al., (1998). Potato carboxypeptidase inhibitor, a T-knot proten, in an epidermal growth factor antagonist that inhibits tumor cell growth. *J. Biol. Chem.*, *273*, 12370-12377.

[24] Frenkel, K., Chrzan, K., Ryan, C. A., et al., (1987). Chymotrypsin – specific protease inhibitors decrease H2O2 formation by activated human polymorphonuclear leukocytes. *Carcinogenesis*, *8*, 1207-1212.

[25] Huang, C. S., Ma, W. Y., Ryan, C. A. & Dong, Z. G. (1997). Proteinase inhibitors I and II from potatoes specifically block UV-induced activator protein-I activation through a pathway that is independent of extracellular signal-regulated kinases, *c*-Jun N-terminal kinases, and p38 kinase. *Proc. Natl. Acad. Sci.*, USA, *94*, 11957-11962.

[26] Melville, J. C. & Ryan, C. A. (1970). Chymotrypsin inhibitor from potatoes : A multisite inhibitor composed of subunits. *Arch. Biochem. Biophys.*, *138*, 700-702.

[27] Brzin, J., Popovic, T., Drobnic-Kosorok, M., et al., (1988). Inhibitors of cysteine proteinases from potato. *Biol. Chem. Hoppe-Seyler*, *369*, suppl., 233-238.

[28] Pouwreau, L., Gruppen, H., Piersma, S. R., et al., (2001). Relative abundance and inhibitory distribution of protease inhibitors in potato juice from Cv. Elkana. *Agric. Food Chem.*, *49*, 2864-2874.

[29] Rozenfel′d, M. A., Leonova, V. B., Biryukova, M. I., Vasil′eva, M. V. & Kostanova, E. A. (1999). Albumin – an inhibitor of fibrinogen aggregation in a solution. *Dokl. Akad. Nauk*, *267(2)*, 269-272.

[30] Lorand, L., Credo, R. B. & Janus, T. J. (1981). Factor XIII (fibrin stabilizing factor). *Method Enzymol.*, *80*, 333-341.

[31] Loewy, A. G. & Dunathan, K. (1961). Fibrinase 1. Purification of substrate and enzyme. *J. Biol. Chem.*, *236*, 2625-2639.

[32] Deutsch, D. G. & Mertz, E. T. (1970). Plasminogen : purification from human plasma by affinity chromatography . *Science*, *170(3962)*, 1095-1099.

[33] Rozenfel′d, M. A., Leonova, V. B., Khavkina, L. S. & Meshkov, B. B. (1984). Antifibrinolytic effect of heparin. *Biochimiya*, *49(10)*, 1672-1678.

[34] Robbins, K. C. & Summaria, L. (1970). Human plasminogen and plasmin. *Method Enzymol.*, *19*, 184-186.

[35] Davies, D. T. & Low, A. J. R. (1977). An improved method for the quantitative fractionation of casein mixtures using ion-exchange chromatography. *J. of Dairy Research*, *44*, 213-221.

[36] Burrett, A. J. (1981). Cystatin, the egg white inhibitor of cysteine proteinases. *Methods Enzymol.*, *80*, 771-778.

[37] Kostanova, E. A., Sokolova, E. V. & Mosolov, V. V. (1986). Description of the composite proteinase sample from the latex of papaya (*Carica papaya*) from the Caucasian Coast of the Black Sea. *Prikl. Biokhim Mikrobiol.*, *22(1)*, 43-48.

[38] Kostanova, E. A., Valueva, T. A., Mosolov, V. V. & Golovkin, B. N. (1988). Comparative study of proteinases from Papaya fruits and leaves. *Prikl. Biokhim. Microbiol.*, *24(6)*, 795-801.

[39] Arnon, R. & Shapira, E., (1968). Antibodies to Papain. A selective fractionation according to inhibitory capacity. *Biochemistry, 6(12)*, 3942-3950.

[40] Laemmli, U. K. (1970). Cleavage of structural proteins during the assembly of the head of bacteriophage T4. *Nature, 227(5259)*, 680-685.

[41] Godal, Y. C., Gravem, K., Brosstad, F. & Nyvold, N. (1984). Quantitation of Factor XIII by SDS polyacrylamide gel electrophoresis *.Thromb. Res., 35*, 577-582.

[42] Marder, V. I., Shulmal, N. R. & Carrol, W. R. (1969). High molecular weight derivatives of human fibrinogen produced by plasmin. *Biol. CHem., 244*, 2111-2119.

[43] Appendorth, K. J. & Augsten, H. (1987). An improvement of the protein determination in plant protein with the dye-binding method according to Bradford. *Biochem. Physiol. Pflanzen., 182(1)*, 85-89.

[44] Doolittle, R. J. (1984). Fibrinogen and Fibrin. *Annu. Rev. Biochem., 53*, 195-229.

[45] Blomback, B. (1996). Fibrinogen and Fibrin – proteins with complex roles in haemostasis and thrombosis. *Thrombos. Res., 83*, 7-75.

[46] Chen, R. & Doolittle, R. J. (1971). γ-γ Crosslinking sites in human and bovine fibrin. *Biochemistry, 10*, 4486-4491.

[47] Pissano, J. J., Finlayson, J. S., Peyton, M. P. & Nayai, J., (1964). ε-(γ-gutamyl)-lysine in fibrin – lack of crosslink formation in Factor XIII deficiency. *Proc.Natl. Acad. Sci.*, USA, *68*, 770-772.

[48] Cooke, R. D. & Holbrook, J. J. (1974). Calcium and the assay of human plasma clotting Factor XIII. *Biochem. J., 141*, 79-84.

[49] Israels, E. D., et al., (1973). Immunological studies of coagulation Factor XIII. *J. Clin. Invest., 52*, 2398-2403.

[50] Lorand, L., et al., (1983). New colored and fluorescent amine substrates for activated fibrin stabilizing factor (FXIIIa) and for transglutaminase. *Arch. Biochem. Biophys., 131*, 419-425.

[51] Gorman, J. J. & Folk, J. E. (1980). Structural features of glutamine substrates for human plasma factor XIIIa (activated blood coagulation factor XIII). *J. Biol. Chem., 255(2)*, 419-427.

In: Human Placenta: Structure and Development... ISBN: 978-1-60876-457-0
Editors: E. Berven, et al. pp. 161-172 © 2010 Nova Science Publishers, Inc.

Chapter VI

Influence of Protein Proteinase Inhibitors to Platelet and Plasma Components of Blood Coagulation

Ya. N. Kotova[1], E.A. Kostanova[2], M.A. Rozenfel'd[2], E.I. Sinauridze[1,3], M. A. Panteleev[1,3] and F. I. Ataullakhanov[1,3,2]*

[1] Center for Theoretical Problems of Physicochemical Pharmacology, Moscow, Russia.
[2] Institute of Biochemical Physics of the Russian Academy fo Sciences.
[3] National Research Center for Hematology, Moscow, Russia.
[4] Lomonosov Moscow State University, Moscow, Russia.

Abstract

Factor XIIIa plays an important role in stabilization of fibrin clot formed during blood coagulation. Recent reports indicate that factor XIIIa influence formation of coated platelets, which have high procoagulant activity and retain on their surface high levels of alphagranule proteins, express surface phosphatidylserine after platelet activation. It was also discovered that new cysteine proteinase inhibitors

* Corresponding author: E-mail: janakoo@yandex.ru

(CPIs) from potato could take regulate factor XIIIa transglutaminase activity. The aim of the present study was to determine the effect of CPIs on coated platelets formation during platelet activation and on enzyme activities in blood coagulation. We found that CPIs decreased the coated platelets subpopulation dose-dependently. They reduced thrombin generation by nearly 40 % both in platelet-rich plasma and in plateletpoor plasma as compared with control, and dose-dependently decreased activity of factor Xa and thrombin. In conclusion, the obtained data show that cysteine proteinase inhibitors have influence on platelet and plasma components of blood coagulation, and suggest that further purification and characterization of these inhibitors are of practical significance and interest.

Keywords: Platelets; Plasma part of blood coagulation; Inhibitors.

Introduction

Coagulation is a complex system of biochemical reactions. Its basic function is prevention of hemorrhage by formation of fibrin clot in case of vessel injury.

The tissue surrounding a vessel (vascular wall), plasma coagulation factors and blood cells (first of all platelets) take part in human hemostatic reaction. The membrane lipid asymmetry disrupts during platelet activation and procoagulant phospholipid phosphatydilserine is exposed in the outer platelet membrane leaflet [1].

Platelet activation leads to appearance of subpopulations that differ in their ability to support coagulation. Activation with thrombin and collagen or with thrombin and convulxin (collagen receptor glycoprotein VI agonist) forms a cell subpopulation termed coated platelets. They retain on their surface high levels of several procoagulant proteins, express phosphatidylserine and support prothrombinase activity [2, 3].

Plasma factor XIII (fibrin stabilizing factor) is a transglutaminase which catalyzes formation of γ-glutamyl-ε-lysin cross links between chains of fibrin molecules. Activated factor XIII (factor XIIIa) plays an important role in stabilization of formed fibrin clot against physical and fibrinolytic damage [4].

It was shown that ~50% of circulating factor XIIIa in blood is contained in platelet cytoplasm [5] and is apparently secreted during platelet activation. Platelet factor XIIIa increases degree of fibrin cross-link and resistance of fibrin to degradation of plasmin [6]. G.L. Dale et al. [3] found that factor XIIIa influences formation of coated platelets. This may suggest a role of this transglutaminase in the increase of procoagulant surface at the site of injury and, therefore, in acceleration of coagulation processes.

Inhibitors of coagulation system are often used for correction of coagulation disorders. It was also discovered that new cysteine proteinase inhibitors (CPIs) from potato could inhibit enzymatic activity of factor XIIIa. The authors were found that these inhibitors possess capability both to modify molecules of fibrin-monomer due to impact on polymerization centers and to affect active site of factor XIIIa that resulted in decrease or absence of crosslinks between fibrin filaments [7].

It should be noted that there are few specific inhibitors of factor XIIIa [8]. The role of platelet factor XIIIa is not clear during platelet activation. This makes development of new inhibitors of plasma and platelet factors XIIIa and investigation of their influence on all parts of coagulation system an important task. The aim of the present study was to determine effects of new cysteine proteinase inhibitors from potato on coated platelets formation during platelet activation and on enzyme activities of plasma coagulation.

Methods

Reagents

The following materials were obtained from the sources shown in brackets: convulxin (Pentapharm, Basel, Switzerland); prostaglandin E1 (MP Biochemicals, Irvine, CA, USA); R-phycoerythrin(PE)- and fluorescein(FITC)- congjugated annexin V (Molecular Probes, Eugene, OR,USA); thromboplastin (Renam, Russia); thrombin (Haematologic Technologies, USA; Roche, France); S2765 (Chromogenix, Italy); fluorogenic substrate BOC-Ile-Gly-Arg-AMC (custom-synthesized at the Institute of Medical and Biological Chemistry RAS, Russia). All other reagents were from Sigma (St Louis, MO, USA).

Cysteine proteinase inhibitors (CPIs) from potato were chosen as described [7].

Obtaining Platelet-Rich and Platelet- Poor Plasma

Blood from healthy donors was collected into 3.8% sodium citrate, pH 5.5, at 9:1 blood/anticoagulant volume ratio. Whole blood was centrifuged at 100 g for 10 min at room temperature to obtain platelet-rich plasma. Whole blood was centrifuged at 1300 g for 15 min at room temperature to obtain platelet- poor plasma.

Platelet Isolation

Platelets were isolated from freshly drawn human blood by centrifugation and gel filtration essentially as described [9]. Briefly, blood was collected into 3.8% sodium citrate, pH 5.5, at 9:1 blood/anticoagulant volume ratio and supplemented with prostaglandin E1 (1 μM) and apyrase (0.1 unit/ml) to prevent activation. Whole blood was centrifuged at 100 g for 10 min at room temperature. The obtained platelet-rich plasma was supplemented with 3.8% sodium citrate, pH 5.5, at 1:3 citrate/plasma ratio to decrease pH. Platelets were concentrated by centrifugation at 400 g for 5 min, resuspended in buffer A (150 mM NaCl, 2.7 mM KCl, 1 mM $MgCl_2$, 0.4 mM NaH_2PO_4, 20 mM HEPES, 5 mM glucose, 0.5% bovine serum albumin) and subjected to gel filtration on a chromatography column packed with Sepharose CL-2B and equilibrated with buffer A.

Determination of Influence of Cysteine Proteinase Inhibitors (CPIs) on Formation of Platelet Heterogeneity

Platelets at 20,000/μl were suspended in buffer A containing 2.5 mM $CaCl_2$. They were stimulated with either thrombin (10nM) or convulxin (100ng/ml) or thrombin (10nM) with convulxin (10ng/ml) with indicated concentrations of CPIs (0; 0.05; 0.1; 0.2; 0.4 mg/ml) for 15 min without stirring and labeled with PE-conjugated or FITC-conjugated annexin V. The samples were immediately analyzed in a FACSCalibur flow cytometer (BD Biosciences). The acquired data were analyzed using a WinMDI 2.8 software (Joseph Trotter, Scripps Research Institute, La Jolla, CA, USA).

Thrombin Generation Assay

Thrombin generation assay was performed according to the basic method of [10, 11] with minor modifications. To wells of 96-well flat bottom plate, 90 μl of platelet poor (PPP), or platelet rich (PRP) citrate plasma, 10 μl of cysteine proteinase inhibitors (CPIs) or buffer (20 mM HEPES, 140 mM NaCl, pH 7.5), and 10 μl of slow fluorogenic substrate BOCIle- Gly-Arg-AMC (5 mM) were added and incubated for 10 min at 37^{0}C. Coagulation was triggered simultaneously in all wells by addition of 25 μl of activator in the same buffer, containing additionally 90 mM $CaCl_2$ (pH 7.5). As activators, 250-fold diluted rabbit thromboplastin solution (PT reagent, Renam, Moscow, Russia) was used. Final concentrations of tissue factor were 4 pM as determined using Actichrome® TF chromogenic activity assay (American Diagnostica, Stamford, CT, USA). AMC fluorescence was monitored continuously for 125-130 min using fluorometric Fluoroscan II reader (LabSystem, Finland) at λ_{ex}=380 nm and λ_{em}=440 nm. Each specimen was reproduced in duplicates, and the mean fluorescence value was used. The data were processed using Origin 6.0 software (Microcal Software, Northampton, MA, USA). Fluorescence intensity was corrected for α_2-macroglobulinthrombin complex activity using a specially written program. Fluorescence was converted to AMC concentration using a calibration determined individually for each sample by measuring fluorescence of a known AMC concentration added to the same plasma with the same CPIs and substrate concentrations. Linearity of the calibration curve under a wide range of AMC concentrations was confirmed in separate experiments (data not shown). From the thrombin generation curve, total area under curve (endogenous thrombin potential (ETP)) for 120 min was determined.

Investigation of the Effect of CPIs on Activity of Thrombin and Factor Xa

Thrombin (10nM) or factor Xa (5 nM) was incubated in buffer A (150 mM NaCl, 2.7 mM KCl, 1 mM $MgCl_2$, 0.4 mM NaH_2PO_4, 20 mM HEPES, 5 mM glucose, 0.5% bovine serum albumin, pH 7.4) with 2.5mM $CaCl_2$. CPIs were added at indicated concentrations (0.05; 0.1; 0.2; 0.4 mg/ml) and incubated for 10 min at 37^{0}C. After that, specific chromogenic substrate for thrombin Chromozym TH or S2765 for factor Xa was added, and initial rate of hydrolysis of the substrate at 405nm for 30min at 37^0C was measured using Thermomax reader (Molecular Devices, USA). The degree of inhibition of each enzyme was estimated as decrease of the rate of hydrolysis (in %) with regard to the rate of hydrolysis in the absence of CPIs, which was assumed to be 100%.

Statistics

The data were compared with the paired Student's t-test. Statistical significance was set as $P < 0.05$. Values are reported as mean ± SE.

Results and Discussion

Influence of ICPs on Coated Platelets Formation

The effect of factor XIIIa on coated platelets formation during platelet activation is not presently clear. In [3], it was found that the presence of factor XIIIa increases this subpopulation whereas [12] suggested that it does not play role in the formation of coated platelets. We can suggest that if factor XIIIa increases coated platelets then it is possible to expect that its inhibitors would influence platelet heterogeneity which appears during cell activation decreasing coated platelets. In our work, we used cysteine proteinase inhibitors (CPIs) from potato which reduce enzymatic activity of factor XIIIa as had been shown earlier [7]. It is necessary to note that preparation of CPIs used in this work was only partially purified and was possibly a mixture several inhibitors containing in initial material. Coated platelets were determined as a cell population with high level of phosphatidylserine on their surface. These cells efficiently bind fluorescently congjugated annexin V. This allows quantitative determination of coated platelets with flow cytometry. The investigation of coated platelets in the presence of different concentrations of CPIs upon activation with various agonists showed that, in all cases, inhibitors dose-dependently decreased coated platelets subpopulation (Figure 1). At maximal concentration of inhibitors (ICPs = 0.4mg/ml) used in experiments, the amount of coated platelets decreased 2- to 10-fold compared with control (ICPs = 0 mg/ml) in the presence of different activators. At that, the half maximum effect was shown at a concentration of ICPs equal to 0.1mg/ml upon dual activation by thrombin with convulxin, whereas upon activation by thrombin or convulxin alone, the half maximum effect was observed at ICPs == 0.05mg/ml. Thus ICPs decrease coated platelets and, therefore, procoagulant surface during coagulation. As we used washed platelets, i.e. plasma proteins were absent from this system, the observed effect of ICPs can be likely explained by influence of inhibitors on platelet factor XIIIa.

Influence of ICPs on Plasma Coagulation

Factor XIII plays an important role in coagulation stabilizing clot by forming cross-link between fibers of polymerizing fibrin. The presence of specific inhibitors of factor XIIIa should not influence processes of thrombin formation during activation of coagulation. Consequently, to characterize possible purity and specificity of ICPs used in this work we studied what influence these inhibitors have on coagulation in plasma.

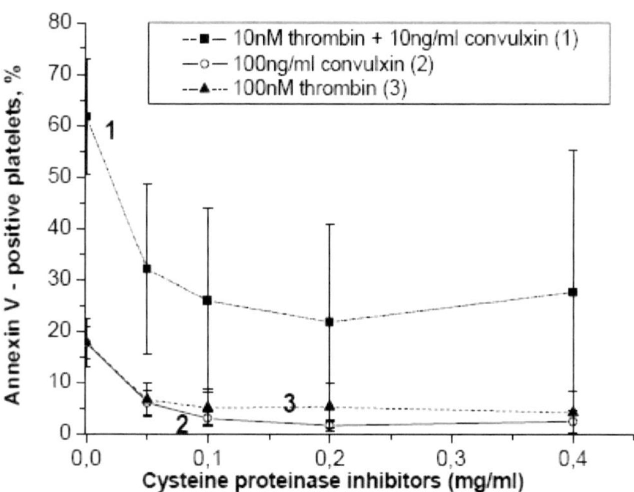

Figure 1. Influence of CPIs on formation of coated platelets. Platelets at 20,000/μl were stimulated with either 1 – thrombin (10nM) or 2 – convulxin (100ng/ml) or 3 – thrombin (10nM) with convulxin (10ng/ml). Mean values±SEM for n=4 experiments with platelets from four donors are shown. P<0.05 for all data.

We used thrombin generation assay (endogenous thrombin potential (ETP)) for description of integral state of system. This test allows characterizing kinetics of thrombin generation and measuring summary quantity of this key coagulation enzyme produced in the sample of plasma in response to standard activation. Thrombin generation was measured in the absence or in the presence of ICPs in both PPP and PRP. Findings are presented Figure 2 and at table. We found that presence of ICPs at a concentration of 0.15 mg/ml decreased ETP by approximately 40% both in PPP and PRP. Also, maximal concentrations of thrombin (A_{max}) were reduced time required to achieve maximal thrombin ($_{tmax}$) and time required to achieve explosive thrombin formation (t_{lag}) were prolonged (see table). Thus, all measurable parameters of thrombin generation assay testified to inhibition of coagulation in the presence of ICPs. Since influence of investigated preparation of inhibitors on ETP was identical in plasmas containing different amounts of platelets, one can suppose that inhibiting influence of ICPs on coagulation is related to inhibiting effect on enzymes of coagulation not on platelets.

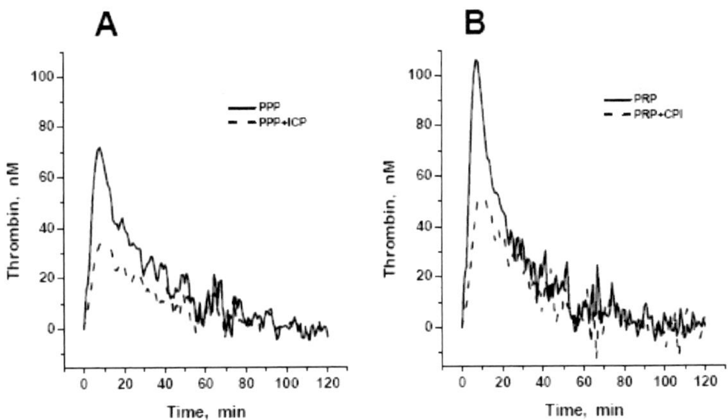

Figure 2. Influence of CPIs (0.15 mg/ml) on values of endogenous thrombin potential in platelet pure (PPP) and platelet rich (PRP) plasma. The typical curves obtained in one of two experiments are shown.

We researched influence of ICPs on activities of thrombin and factor Xa in purified buffer system with specific chromogenic substrates to revealing points of possible effect of inhibitors in coagulation. The findings are shown in Figure 3. In both cases, ICPs dose-dependently decreased activities of these enzymes. Inhibition of thrombin was 10% at maximum concentration of ICPs

(0.4mg/ml) and was not significantly different whereas inhibition of factor Xa was about 30% and significantly different (Figure 3). As activated factor Xa is a member of prothrombinase complex, its and may be cause of ETP decrease in the presence of ICPs.

Table. Influence of CPIs on thrombin generation

Sample*)	ETP, nM*min	t_{max}, min	A_{max}, nM	$t_{5nM,}$ min	Decrease ETP, %
PPP	2027.6	7.93	71.88	0.39	–
PPP + CPIs	1165.7	8.88	34.33	0.78	42.5
(0.154 mg/ml)					
PRP	2355.3	6.97	106.05	0.33	–
PRP + CPIs	1437.2	10.75	51.07	0.78	39.0
(0.150 mg/ml)					

*) PPP – platelet poor plasma, PRP – platelet rich plasma.

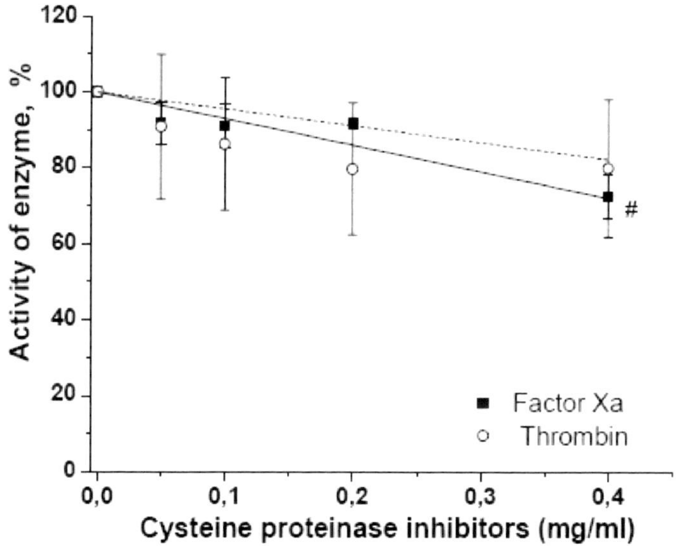

Figure 3. Decrease of activities of thrombin and factor Xa in the presence of different concentrations of CPIs. The reactions were carried out in buffer systems in the presence of specific chromogenic substrates. Mean values±SEM for n=4 experiments. # $P<0.05$, for data of factor Xa.

Influence of ICPs on thrombin generation supposes that these inhibitors could act not only on factor Xa and thrombin, but also on other procoagulant factors of coagulation, for example, on activity of extrinsic tenase. All this needs further study.

Consequently, we found that ICPs from potato, on the one hand, decrease activity of platelet factor XIIIa and, on the other hand, reduce coated platelets formation. The findings can have great practical significance as there are few inhibitors of factor XIIIa, and they are not for clinical use. Increased activity of factor XIIIa is associated with numerous pathologies. It is observed in patients with thromboembolic complications, atherosclerosis, pancreatic diabetes, etc. [13, 14]. Higher activity of factor XIIIa can be a risk factor leading to thrombosis, and it can be a promising target for therapeutic inhibition. However, as investigated ICPs are not completely separated yet, now and for identification of their specificity and toxicity requires further purification and research.

Acknowledgments

The study was supported by Russian Academy of Sciences Presidium Basic Research Programs 'Molecular and Cellular Biology' (MCB RAS Russia) and 'Basic Sciences for Medicine', by Russian Foundation for Basic Research grants 07-04-00146, 08-04-12060, 09-04-00232, 09-04-00357 and 09-04-92427, and by Russian Federation President Grant for Young Scientists MK-340.2008.4.

References

[1] Zwaal, R. F. A. & Schroit, A. J. (1997). Pathophysiologic implications of membrane phospholipids asymmetry in blood cells. *Blood*, *Vol. 89 №4*, 1121-1132.

[2] Alberio, L., Safa, O., Clemetson, K. J., Esmon, C. T. & Dale, G. L. (2000). Surface expression and functional characterization of ⟨-granule factorV in human platelets: effect of ionophore A23187, thrombin, collagen, and convulxin. *Blood*, *Vol. 95*, 1694-1702.

[3] Dale, G. L., Friese, P., Batar, P., Hamilton, S. F., Reed, G. L., Jackson, K. W., Clemetson, K. J. & Alberio, L. (2002). Stimulated platelets use serotonin to enhance their retention of procoagulant proteins on the cell surface. *Nature*, *Vol. 415*, 175-179.

[4] Sane, D. C., Kontos, J. L. & Greenberg, C. S. (2007). Roles of transglutaminases in cardiac and vascular diseases. *Bioscience*, *Vol. 12*, 2530-2545.

[5] Serrano, K. & Devine, D. V. (2002). Intracellular factor XIII crosslinks platelet cyto skeletal elements upon platelet activation. *Thromb Haemost*, *Vol. 88*, 315-320.

[6] Greenberg, C. S., Birckbichler, P. J. & Rice, R. H. (1991). Transglutaminases: multifunctional cross-linking enzymes that stabilize tissues. *FASEB J.*, *Vol. 5*, 3071-3077.

[7] Kostanova, E. A., Rozenfel'd, M. A., Revina, T. A. & Valueva, T. A. (2007). Protein inhibitors of fibrin stabilizing factor FXIII. *Izv Akad Nauk Ser Biol.*, *Vol. 3*, 28283-28289.

[8] Sugimura, Y., Hosono, M., Wada, F., Yoshimura, T., Maki, M. & Hitomi, K. (2006). Screening for the preferred substrate sequence of transglutaminase using a phage-displayed peptide library. Identification of peptide substrates for TGase2 and factor XIIIA. *J. Biol. Chem.*, *Vol. 281 №26*, 17699-17706.

[9] Panteleev, M. A., Ananyeva, N. M., Greco, N. J., Ataullakhanov, F. I. & Saenko, E. L. (2005). Two subpopulations of thrombin-activated platelets differ in their binding of the components of the intrinsic factor Xactivating complex. *J Thromb Haemost*, *Vol. 3*, 2545-2553.

[10] Hemker, H. C., Giesen, P. L. A., Ramjee, M., Wagenvoord, R. & Beguin, S. (2000). The thrombogram: Monitoring thrombin generation in platelet rich plasma. *Thromb. Haemost.*, *Vol. 83 №4*, 589-591.

[11] Hemker, H. C., Giesen, P. L. A., AlDieri, R., Regnault, V., de Smed, E., Wagenvoord, R., Lecompte, T. & Beguin, S. (2002). The Calibrated Automated Thrombogram (CAT): a universal routine test for hyper- and hypocoagulability. *Pathophysiol. Haemost. Thromb.*, *Vol. 32 №5-6*, 249-253.

[12] Jobe, S. M., Leo, L., Eastvold, J. S., Dickeneite, G., Ratliff, T. L., Lentz, S. R. & Paola, J. D. (2005). Role of FcRg and factor XIIIA in coated platelet formation. *Blood*, *Vol. 106*, 4146-4151.

[13] Kohler, H. P. (2001). Role of blood coagulation factor XIII in vascular disease. *Swiss Med Wkly*, *Vol. 131*, 31-34.

[14] Ametov, A. S. & Kondrat'eva, L. V. (2006). Metaformin – basic of therapy patient with metabolic syndrome. *Endocrinology*, *Vol. 14 № 26*, 1905-1911.

In: Human Placenta: Structure and Development... ISBN: 978-1-60876-457-0
Editors: E. Berven, et al. pp. 173-180 © 2010 Nova Science Publishers, Inc.

Chapter VII

Predicting Development and Disease in Infancy and Childhood from Placental Function

Jörg Dötsch[1*], Regina Trollmann[1], Anja Tzschoppe[1], Ellen Struwe[1] and Ralf Schild[2]

[1]Department of Pediatrics, University Hospital Erlangen.

[2]Diakonische Dienste, Hannover.

Summary

Placenta and fetus are closely linked in the so-called feto-placental unit. Therefore, the placenta contains information of intrauterine fetal life. This information might be of relevance for future processes in the then independent human organism. There are two principle ways of getting access to placental endocrine function with relevance for the fetus. More indirectly, during pregnancy serological maternal examinations e.g. of angiogenetic factors may help to predict the risk of evolving preeclampsia and possible secondary fetal involvement. However, direct access to the fetal side of the feto-placental unit is more difficult without injury at least during pregnancy. After delivery there is easy availability of placental samples, allowing for the analysis of feto-placental endocrinology and potential prediction of future developments

* Corresponding author: Department of Pediatrics, University Hospital Erlangen, Loschgestr. 15, 91054 Erlangen, Germany, E-mail: Joerg.Doetsch@uk-erlangen.de

arising from these conditions. We are currently conducting a multicenter study to predict the probability of later disease inflicted by a hostile intrauterine environment. An early prediction of risk of future disease would help to initiate early preventive measures.

Keywords: Endocrine regulation, placenta, prediction, fetal programming.

Introduction

Throughout human history the afterbirth (placenta) has raised many questions. Even today we are only gradually gaining knowledge of the function and dysfunction of such a complex organ that is needed for a relatively short period of time in life, i.e. from shortly after conception until birth. However, is the role of the placenta definitely ending with birth and expulsion from the maternal womb? Or do the placenta and its "ingredients" play another role after childbirth? Does the placenta bear signals for an individual's future? Mankind has repeatedly searched for a solution to this question, mostly by the help of religion and mysticism. On the other hand, in the last decades the search for scientific solutions to these questions has started.

Mystical Role of the Afterbirth

It has been known from one of the first high cultures of mankind that events associated with birth were interpreted as hidden or overt divine signals. For instance, Siamese twins or short statured newborns were associated with goddesses (Cozma, 2006). The afterbirth was even more mysterious: Its physiological role was obscure at that time. It was thought that parts of the human soul survived in placental tissue, giving rise to the ceremonial of placental burial (Murray, 1930). Traditions of ceremonial burial of the placenta are known from various cultures around the world throughout history. They were reported from China, ancient Palestine, the Aborigines in Australia and from Europe.

It was not before the 18th century that the unit between mother, placenta and fetus started to be understood (John Hunter 1718-1793). Its exact role in the transport of oxygen, nutrients, and waste products was, however, not understood until the 20th century.

Can the Feto-Placental Unit and the Placenta Predict a Newborn´s Future?

From a scientific point of view the close interaction between placenta and fetus has been proven conclusively (Osada et al., 2002, Constância et al., 2002). Therefore, fetus and placenta may be regarded as one closely interrelated unit, sending messages from placenta to fetus and vice-versa. To ensure synergy between fetus and placenta, signals would have to be sensed by both systems in a similar way. As a consequence, environmental changes leading to persistent alterations in the fetus should be reflected in the placenta as well. Fetal tissue is not available for further analysis. In contrary, the placenta is completely accessible for analysis. Theoretically, the placenta might be the mirror of essential, long standing changes for the newborn baby's later health, a concept that is also called "fetal programming of adult disease".

Prediction of Disease after Short Term Oxygen Deprivation (Prenatal Asphyxia) (Figure 1)

Prenatal oxygen deprivation to the fetus (asphyxia) is one of the most feared birth complications. Consequences of perinatal asphyxia are temporary or persistent cerebral alterations, called hypoxic ischemic encephalopathy (HIE). While the least severe degree (HIE I) only lasts for several hours to days the most severe grade (HIE III) leads to sequelae such as cerebral palsy throughout life (Khot et al., 2006). To date, there are no parameters at birth which allow a reliable prediction of outcome after asphyxia. In view of the ever increasing therapeutic options, a prediction of the outcome is of paramount importance (Jacobs et al., 2007). As the placenta is the organ transporting oxygen from the mother to her fetus it appears logical that it will at least partly suffer from the same degree of oxygen deprivation.

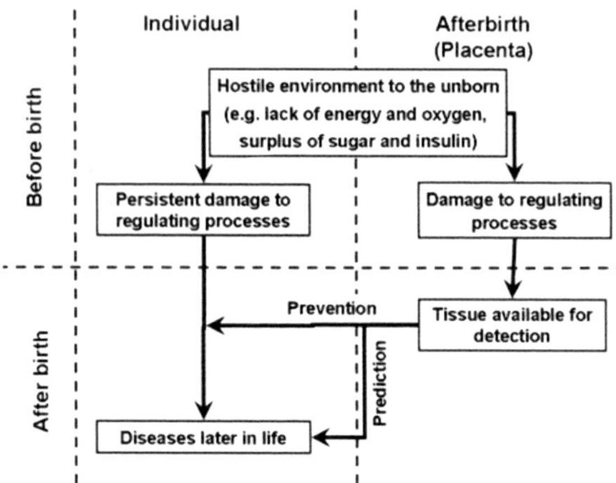

Figure 1. Concept of prediction of diseases later in life on the basis of the so-called feto-placental unit: Adverse environmental conditions to the unborn child (fetus) are prevalent in the placenta and the fetus at the same time. Disease-predisposing alterations in the fetus are therefore reflected by the placenta. Placental tissue is available for the detection of these changes (while fetal tissue is certainly not). Detection of these changes allows a prediction of later disease and (more importantly) of early prevention.

Oxygen deprivation leads to the activation of several mechanisms to counteract its harmful consequences. Among these are synthesis of substances promoting the growth of new blood vessels and agents leading to an opening (dilatation) of blood vessels supplying the area of low oxygen tension. It was recently shown that two of these factors in the placenta (adrenomedullin and vascular endothelial growth factor) can predict whether an infant will suffer from the most severe form of prenatal oxygen deprivation bearing the risk of cerebral palsy later in life (Trollmann et al., 2002, 2003, 2007). Therefore, early determination of these and other factors in the placenta may allow for an early identification of newborn babies with the highest risk permitting an early commencement of adequate treatment.

Alterations of the Fetal Environment and Disease Later in Life

A frequent fetal complication during fetal life is intrauterine growth restriction (IUGR). For a number of years already, predictors for evolving

IUGR have been successfully described (Ness et al., 2007; Thame et al., 2001). Especially preeclampsia, as the most important maternal disease during pregnancy can in parts been foreseen by adequate laboratory tests e.g. by measuring angiogenetic factors in maternal serum or urine (Moore Simas et al., 2007; Aggarwal et al., 2006). With regard to the fetus, it is of special interest that not only preeclampsia but also the extend of the associated IUGR can be predicted (Chafetz et al., 2007).

While the concept of long term diseases caused by a hostile fetal environment is not new (Dörner et al., 1988), its impact has come to wider attention with the observation that intrauterine starvation as in low birth weight is associated with a higher risk of myocardial infarction later in life (Barker et al., 1989). Similar observations were for instance made for the association of low birth weight and diabetes mellitus type 2 and overweight. While research is meanwhile focussing on potential mechanisms of these associations and others, there is one major question from a newborn individual's perspective: Am I at risk for developing a disease that is associated with my adverse intrauterine environment or not? Could I profit from a close monitoring of my health status? Are there options to prevent potential disease (Figure 1)?

Albeit being predominantly at risk for a certain disease in adult life after having been exposed to an adverse intrauterine environment, alterations of essential regulatory processes may already be present in children as young as 4-6 years of age: Children who had a low birth weight already showed signs of overweight or even changes predisposing to later diabetes mellitus (Ibañez et al., 2006). It is, however, still unknown whether the newborn baby will indeed suffer from a higher probability of development of these diseases later in life.

Prediction of Later Disease by Analysis of the Placenta?

Based on the concept of the feto-placental unit we designed a controlled multicenter study aiming at predicting later disease by analysing the placenta right after birth. In the placenta of infants suffering from intrauterine nutrient deprivation resulting in diminished growth in the womb important regulating systems (systems important for cell growth and transport through the placenta) are analysed by different methods (determination of gene expression and protein concentration). All essential perinatal data are collected after the parents have been asked for informed written consent.

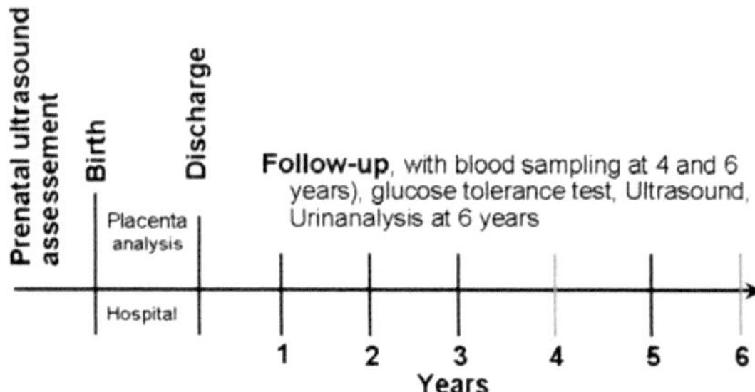

Figure 2. Schematic outline of the FIPS (Fetal programming-intrauterine growth restriction-placenta-study). It is the aim of the study to predict the probability of long term disease after intrauterine nutrient deprivation by analysing placental regulatory systems and relating them to clinical follow-up examinations.

In the following 6 years the patients will be examined annually with regard to growth, overweight, blood pressure, kidney function, and glucose tolerance (Figure 2). The data are then related to placental regulating systems that may have been altered during intrauterine nutrient deprivation. It will have to be seen whether certain markers turn out to be predictive of the child's later health. One first hint at the potential usefulness of this concept is the observation that the enzyme 11β-hydroxysteroid dehydrogenase type 2 (that converts active cortisol into inactive cortisone) is inversely correlated with growth velocity in the first year of life after IUGR (Tzschoppe et al., in press).

Conclusions

Although there is no indication that the placenta hosts anything essential of the newborn baby (as believed by various cultures before introduction of modern medicine) the information the placenta has stored as a mirror of intrauterine life may reflect future disease-predisposing changes. An early revelation of the placenta´s biochemical secrets might therefore help to prevent certain disease in later life.

References

[1] Kozma, C. Dwarfs in ancient Egypt. *Am J Med Genet A.*, 2006, 15, 140, 303-11.

[2] Murray, MA. The bundle of life. 1930. *Ancient Egypt III*, 65-73.

[3] Osada, H; Watanabe, Y; Nishimura, Y; Yukawa, M; Seki, K; Sekiya, S. Profile of trace element concentrations in the feto-placental unit in relation to fetal growth. *Acta Obstet Gynecol Scand*, 2002, 81, 931-7.

[4] Constância, M; Hemberger, M; Hughes, J; Dean, W; Ferguson-Smith, A; Fundele, R; Stewart, F; Kelsey, G; Fowden, A; Sibley, C; Reik, W. Placental-specific IGF-II is a major modulator of placental and fetal growth. *Nature*, 2002, 27, 417, 945-8.

[5] Trollmann, R; Klingmüller, K; Schild, RL; Rascher, W; Dötsch, J. Differential gene expression of somatotrophic and growth factors in response to in vivo hypoxia in human placenta. *Am J Obstet Gynecol.*, 2007, 197, 601.e1-6.

[6] Trollmann, R; Amann, K; Schoof, E; Beinder, E; Wenzel, D; Rascher, W; Dötsch, J. Hypoxia activates the human placental vascular endothelial growth factor system in vitro and in vivo: up-regulation of vascular endothelial growth factor in clinically relevant hypoxic ischemia in birth asphyxia. *Am J Obstet Gynecol.*, 2003, 188, 517-23.

[7] Khot, S; Tirschwell, DL. Long-term neurological complications after hypoxic-ischemic encephalopathy. *Semin Neurol.*, 2006, 26, 422-31.

[8] Jacobs, S; Hunt, R; Tarnow-Mordi, W; Inder, T; Davis, P. Cooling for newborns with hypoxic ischaemic encephalopathy. *Cochrane Database Syst Rev.*, 2007, 17, CD003311.

[9] Trollmann, R; Schoof, E; Beinder, E; Wenzel, D; Rascher, W; Dötsch, J. Adrenomedullin gene expression in human placental tissue and leukocytes: a potential marker of severe tissue hypoxia in neonates with birth asphyxia. *Eur J Endocrinol.*, 2002, 147, 711-6.

[10] Ness, RB; Bass, D; Hill, L; Klebanoff, MA; Zhang, J. Diagnostic test characteristics of placental weight in the prediction of small-for-gestational-age neonates. *J Reprod Med.*, 2007, 52, 793-800.

[11] Thame, M; Osmond, C; Wilks, R; Bennett, FI; Forrester, TE. Second-trimester placental volume and infant size at birth. *Obstet G ynecol.*, 2001, 98, 279-83.

[12] Moore Simas, TA; Crawford, SL; Solitro, MJ; Frost, SC; Meyer, BA; Maynard, SE. Angiogenic factors for the prediction of preeclampsia in high-risk women. *Am J Obstet Gynecol.*, 2007, 197, 244.e1-8.

[13] Aggarwal, PK; Jain, V; Sakhuja, V; Karumanchi, SA; Jha, V. Low urinary placental growth factor is a marker of pre-eclampsia. *Kidney Int.*, 2006, 69, 621-4.

[14] Chafetz, I; Kuhnreich, I; Sammar, M; Tal, Y; Gibor, Y; Meiri, H; Cuckle, H; Wolf, M. First-trimester placental protein 13 screening for preeclampsia and intrauterine growth restriction. *Am J Obstet Gynecol.*, 2007, 197, 35.e1-7.

[15] Tjoa, ML; Oudejans, CB; van Vugt, JM; Blankenstein, MA; van Wijk, IJ. Markers for presymptomatic prediction of preeclampsia and intrauterine growth restriction. *Hypertens Pregnancy*, 2004, 23, 171-89.

[16] Dörner, G; Plagemann, A; Rückert, J; Götz, F; Rohde, W; Stahl, F; Kürschner, U; Gottschalk, J; Mohnike, A; Steindel, E. Teratogenetic maternofoetal transmission and prevention of diabetes susceptibility. *Exp Clin Endocrinol.*, 1988, 91, 247-58.

[17] Barker, DJ; Winter, PD; Osmond, C; Margetts, B; Simmonds, SJ. Weight in infancy and death from ischaemic heart disease. *Lancet*, 1989, 2, 577-80

[18] Ibáñez, L; Ong, K; Dunger, DB; de Zegher, F. Early development of adiposity and insulin resistance after catch-up weight gain in small-for-gestational-age children. *J Clin Endocrinol Metab.*, 2006, 91, 2153-8.

[19] Tzschoppe, A; Struwe, E; Blessing, H; Fahlbusch, F; Liebhaber, G; Dörr, HG; Rauh, M; Rascher, W; Goecke, TW; Schild, RL; Schleussner, E; Scheler, C; Hübler, A; Dahlem, P; Dötsch, J. Placental 11ß-HSD2 gene expression at birth is inversely correlated with growth velocity in the first year of life after intrauterine growth restriction (IUGR). *Ped. Res.*, In press.

In: Human Placenta: Structure and Development... ISBN: 978-1-60876-457-0
Editors: E. Berven, et al. pp. 181-212 © 2010 Nova Science Publishers, Inc.

Chapter VIII

The Activity of Angiotensin II in the Human Placenta

Gershon Holcberg [1,3]***, Alaa Amash*** [2,3]***, Olga Sapir*** [1,3]***,***
Eyal Sheiner [1,3] ***and Mahmoud Huleihel*** [2,3]

[1]Department of Obstetrics and Gynecology, Soroka University Medical Center, Beer Sheva, Israel.

[2]The Shraga Segal Department of Microbiology and Immunology, Beer Sheva, Israel.

[3]Faculty of Health Sciences, Ben-Gurion University of the Negev, Beer Sheva, Israel.

Abstract

The renin-angiotensin system (RAS) is one of main regulators of blood pressure and electrolyte balance during pregnancy. All the components of the RAS have been reported to be expressed in the utero-placental unit. Angiotensin (Ang) II is increasingly recognized as a growth factor, both in its own right and through interactions with other growth factors. Ang II synthesized in the placenta may serve as an autocrine/paracrine modulator of placental function. In addition to its role in regulation of blood pressure during normal pregnancy, Ang II is suggested to be involved in regulation of placentation through regulation of trophoblast invasion, angiogenesis and placental vascular development. These key effects of Ang II, in addition to its capacity to induce inflammatory response, suggest that increased vascular sensitivity to Ang II may have an important role in the increase in vascular resistance and elevated blood pressure seen pregnancy complications such as intra-uterin growth retardation (IUGR) and preeclampsia. Magnesium sulfate ($MgSO_4$) is used in pregnancy as either prophylaxis/treatment for eclamptic seizures or for preterm labor tocolysis. Our group has shown that $MgSO_4$ may attenuate Ang II induced placental vasoconstriction, and may affect Ang II induced placental cytokine production. This review summarizes the current understanding of the physiological aspects of Ang II in the utero-placental unit and its role in the pathogenesis of pregnancy disorders such as preeclampsia. Furthermore, the possible interactions between Ang II and $MgSO_4$ in the placental unit are also discussed.

1. Introduction

The renin-angiotensin system (RAS) is a signaling cascade that plays a key role in regulating blood pressure and electrolyte balance. The reaction between renin, an aspartyl protease and its substrate, angiotensinogen, is the initial and rate-limiting step of this enzymatic cascade that generates the decapeptide angiotensin (Ang) I. Ang I is further processed to the most potent vasoactive octapeptide Ang II by angiotensin-converting enzyme (ACE) [1].

Traditionally, the RAS has been considered primarily as a circulating system involved in the regulation of blood pressure and salt and fluid homeostasis. In addition to this classic view of the RAS, accumulating evidence indicates that the components of the RAS are synthesized in many tissues, such as brain, heart, ovary, and placenta, and that Ang II levels can be controlled locally, independent of circulating Ang II [2-3]. These local RASs may function independently or in concert with the circulating RAS and participate in a paracrine and autocrine regulation of various aspects of tissue function.

Ang II is responsible for most of the physiological and pathophysiological effects of the RAS. It is not just a potent vasopressor which raises systemic blood pressure but it also mediates a broad array of physiological and pathophysiological effects by binding to specific cell membrane receptors. Two distinct types of G-protein-coupled receptors for Ang II have been cloned and characterized in humans and rodents. The angiotensin type 1 (AT1) receptor is predominantly expressed in the kidneys, adrenal glands, vascular smooth muscle cells and the heart. The regulatory actions of Ang II on blood pressure and salt/water balance have been attributed to this receptor [4-6]. The

AT2 receptor is present at high density during fetal development, while in the adult, significant AT2 receptor expression occurs only in the adrenal medulla, uterus, ovary, vascular endothelium, adrenal glands and certain areas in the brain [7-8]. The AT2 receptor is thought to counterbalance effects mediated by the AT1 receptor: it appears to induce vasodilatation and may be involved in the control of cell proliferation, differentiation and angiogenesis [5,7-8].

2. Angiotensin II in the Utero-Placental Unit

The expression and localization of all RAS components in the utero-placental unite are well studied and defined. Renin is presented by all parts of the human utero-placental unit, with highest renin levels in the fetal membranes and the decidua [9]. The expression of renin mRNA by human placenta indicates the potential local renin synthesis [10]. Angiotensinogen peptide and mRNA were also found in the human placenta [10-12]. Moreover, expression and high activity of ACE were reported in the human uterus, placenta and fetal membranes [13-14].

The examination of ACE localization in the placenta directly revealed that ACE mRNA is localized primarily in vessel fraction of the placenta, especially in venous endothelial cells of stem villous of the placenta [15]. The ACE activity in vessel fractions is significantly higher than those in other fractions of the placenta. Moreover, the ACE activity of umbilical venous endothelial cells is significantly higher than that of umbilical arterial endothelial cells, suggesting that the placental and umbilical venous endothelial cells would be the main site for the conversion of Ang I to Ang II.

Ang II receptors of both AT1 and AT2 were demonstrated in placentas and fetal membranes of humans and other species [16]. The AT1 receptors are the predominant receptors in the human placenta [17-18], and are localized in the cytotrophoblast and syncytiotrophoblasts in the placental villi, in extravillous trophoblast, and around the blood vessels of the placental villi [18-19].

The presence of cathepsin D and chymase in the uterus indicates that alternative pathways for Ang II generation may exist independent from renin and ACE [20-21]. The placenta is known to produce large amounts of enzymes capable of Ang II degradation [22], such as aminopeptidase A produced in the fetal placenta which can degrade locally generated Ang II and thus may act as an effective barrier for Ang II between the fetoplacental and the maternal intervillous circulations [23].

The conditions for Ang II formation exist and Ang II receptors are present throughout the human utero-placental unit, indicating the presence of a functional local RAS. These findings also suggest that Ang II synthesized in the placenta may serve as an autocrine/paracrine modulator of placental function.

3. Physiological Aspects of Angiotensin II in the Utero-Placental Unit

3.1. Regulation of the Utero-Placental Vascular Resistance and Blood Flow

The primary function of the placenta is to act as an interface between mother and fetus that allows, and even promotes, fetal growth and development, and to contribute to the maternal cardiovascular adaptations of pregnancy. Appropriate perfusion of the placenta is necessary for its critical endocrine and exchange functions. The regulation of vascular resistance and blood flow in the utero-placental unit is complex [24]. As this circulation is not innervated, vascular tone and resistance to blood flow must be largely controlled by autocrine or paracrine factors [25]. One of the postulated mechanisms by which the placenta may influence maternal vascular tone is the placental RAS.

In human pregnancy, on the maternal side of utero-placental unit, there are two major renin-producing circulations, namely, renal circulation and utero-placental circulation. Experimentally, in pregnant rabbits, a reciprocal relationship between uterine and renal renin synthesis has been demonstrated; i.e., when uterine renin synthesis is increased, renal renin synthesis is reciprocally decreased [26]. A complete local tissue-based RAS in the utero-placental unit may regulate the regional maternal intervillous blood flow [27].

The maternal circulating RAS and utero-placental tissue RAS has been thought to support maternal placental flow by raising maternal arterial pressure or changing placental vascular resistance. Previously, our group has examined the vasoactive effect of Ang II on uncomplicated human perfused placenta, and showed that bolus injections of Ang II (10^{-9}–10^{-5} M) resulted in a significant increase in perfusion pressure in a dose-dependent manner as compared with basal pressure, indicating that Ang II is a possible regulator of placental blood flow during pregnancy (Figure 1) [28].

The placenta or uterus may alter maternal circulating RAS. During normal pregnancy, plasma renin concentration, renin activity, and Ang II levels are elevated. However, the vascular responsiveness to Ang II appears to be reduced [29-30]. The systemic vasculature is thus refractory to Ang II in normal pregnancy, i.e., requires a higher Ang II infusion rate (almost twice as high compared with nongravid at the peak refractory state) for the same degree of vascular response [31-32]. This vascular refractoriness to Ang II in pregnancy has been ascribed, in part, to progesterone and prostacycline [33]. Angiotensinogen levels also increase in pregnancy, but the exact timing of this change is not well defined. Aldosterone levels are increased, and this may contribute to sodium retention and resultant obligatory water retention, which is one of the mechanisms of volume expansion in pregnancy [34].

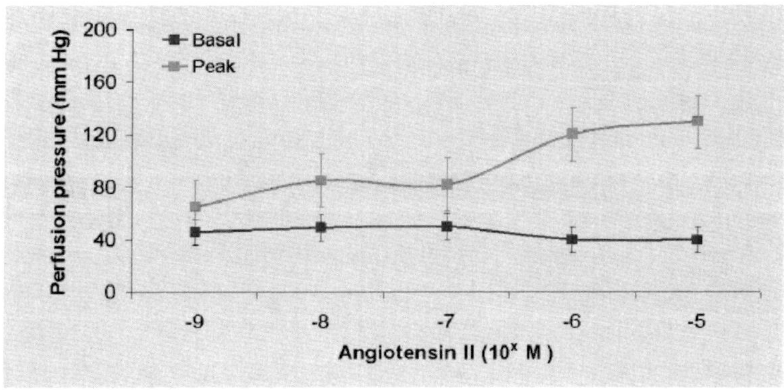

Figure 1. Pressor response to Ang II in an isolated placental cotyledon from a normal placenta.

The control of vascular tone and blood pressure achieved by Ang II is probably mediated by vascular endothelial synthesis of prostaglandins. The vascular response to Ang II has been shown to be diminished by the use of prostaglandin inhibitors, indomethacin and aspirin [35-36]. During normal pregnancy there is an increased production of the potent vasodilator prostacyclin, and the vasoconstrictor thromboxane A_2, with a delicate balance which favors prostacyclin [37]. Our group has also shown that the vasoconstrictor effect of Ang II on feto-placental vasculator is attenuated by atrial natriuretic peptide (ANP) and brain natriuretic peptide (BNP) [38].

3.2. Implantation and Placentation

Ang II is increasingly recognized as a growth factor, independently and through interactions with other growth factors. In addition to its well-known effects on the cardiovascular system and on salt and water homeostasis, Ang II through its AT1 receptor also mediates processes that are likely to be important for successful placentation, including cellular proliferation and growth [39] and angiogenesis [40-41]. The AT1 receptor is present in the placenta throughout pregnancy [42] and has been localized to cytotrophoblast, syncytiotrophoblast, extravillous trophoblast and perivascular cells [43].

Trophoblast invasion, implantation and placental development depend, in part, on the controlled production of plasmin from plasminogen, a process regulated by plasminogen activators (PAs) and plasminogen activator inhibitors (PAIs) [44-45]. Ang II, through the AT1 receptor, has been shown to regulate plasminogen activation through stimulation of PAI-1 synthesis and secretion in human trophoblasts [46]. Moreover, activation of the RAS may induce multiple growth factors that have been implicated in fibrosis, such as transforming growth factor-β (TGF-β) and platelet-derived growth factor-β (PDGF-β) [47-49]. Induction of these growth factors is mediated by Ang II action on the AT1 receptor [50]. TGF-β1 inhibits trophoblast invasion [51], proliferation [52], migration [53], and limits degradation of the extracellular matrix by extravillous trophoblast [52]. Since TGF-β1 is produced predominantly by the maternal decidua, it may provide a mechanism to prevent over-invasion.

Furthermore, all RAS components also exist in the maternal placenta, i.e., the decidua. The decidua has been shown to be a major source of renin in the gravid human uterus [54]. Angiotensinogen, renin, ACE, and AT1 are expressed in and around the spiral arteries of the first-trimester decidua [55]. Moreover, renin and angiotensinogen expression has been also described in prolactin-producing human decidual cells from the third trimester of pregnancy [56]. The molecular evidence of a tissue-based RAS in the decidua may have several implications: The local spiral artery RAS may play a role in the pregnancy-associated vascular modeling of the spiral arteries [57]. The synthesis of renin and angiotensinogen in the prolactin-producing endocrine cells of the decidua has implications for the regulation of this RAS [56]. Transformation of uterine-lining endometrial stromal cells to the decidual cells of pregnancy and expression and secretion of prolactin are regulated by estrogen, progesterone, and several other paracrine factors [58]. The sex steroids also regulate hepatic angiotensinogen expression [59]. Therefore, decidual RAS may be regulated by estrogen and progesterone and by other factors involved in decidualization [56]. Progesterone treatment of decidual cells or endometrial stromal cells in vitro increases active renin secretion [60-61]. Uterine renin secretion is a constitutive secretion, with a response time of hours for various stimuli compared with renal renin, which has a regulated secretion, cells having storage granules and a response time of few minutes [62].

Additional important growth factor in placental development is the vascular endothelial growth factor (VEGF) family and their receptors. VEGF is expressed in the placenta by villous trophoblasts in the first trimester, by extravillous trophoblasts at term and by both fetal and maternal macrophages [63]. There are two receptors for VEGF, VEGF-R1, also known as fms-like tyrosine kinase (or Flt-1) and kinase domain receptor (VEGF-R2). Ang II induces angiogenesis in several in vivo models [40,64-66], including the chroioallantoic membrane assay [66] and the corneal pocket model of the rabbit [40]. Ang II infusion increases capillary density in several animal models [40,65-66]. Ang II has several stimulatory effects on angiogenesis including the induction of VEGF [67-68], hypoxia-inducible factor (HIF)-1α [69], and VEGFR-2 [70] expression. The proangiogenic effects of Ang II appear to be mediated by the AT1 receptor [65,71-72]. Ang II can also act at the AT2 receptor and activation of the AT2 receptor has been reported to have an inhibitory effect on angiogenesis. Ang II has been reported to inhibit VEGF mediated tube formation by endothelial cells through AT2 activation [73].

Towards the end of gestation, continued placental vascular development is terminated, a process accomplished in part through the production of antiangiogenic factors. One such antiangiogenic factor is a soluble form of VEGFR-1 (sFlt-1) that binds to circulating VEGF and placental growth factor, thereby inhibiting their angiogenic activities. sFlt-1, a vascular growth factor antagonist produced by the placenta, is released into the maternal circulation [74]. Infusion of Ang II has been shown to increase circulating levels of sFlt-1 in pregnant mice, demonstrating that Ang II is a regulator of sFlt-1 secretion in vivo. Furthermore, Ang II stimulated sFlt-1 production by human villous explants and cultured trophoblasts but not by endothelial cells, suggesting that trophoblasts are the primary source of sFlt-1 during pregnancy.

In summary, Ang II is one of the key factors regulating the process of placentation through regulation of trophoblast invasion, angiogenesis and placental vascular development.

4. The Role of Angiotensin II in Preeclampsia

The fact that the RAS is one of the main regulators of vascular resistance and blood flow during pregnancy suggests that disruptions in this system may play a critical role in pregnancy disorders. Several indirect lines of evidence indicate that the up-regulation of RAS in the placenta might be important for the pathogenesis of some clinical disorders, such as pregnancy-associated hypertension (PAH) and preeclampsia [75-77].

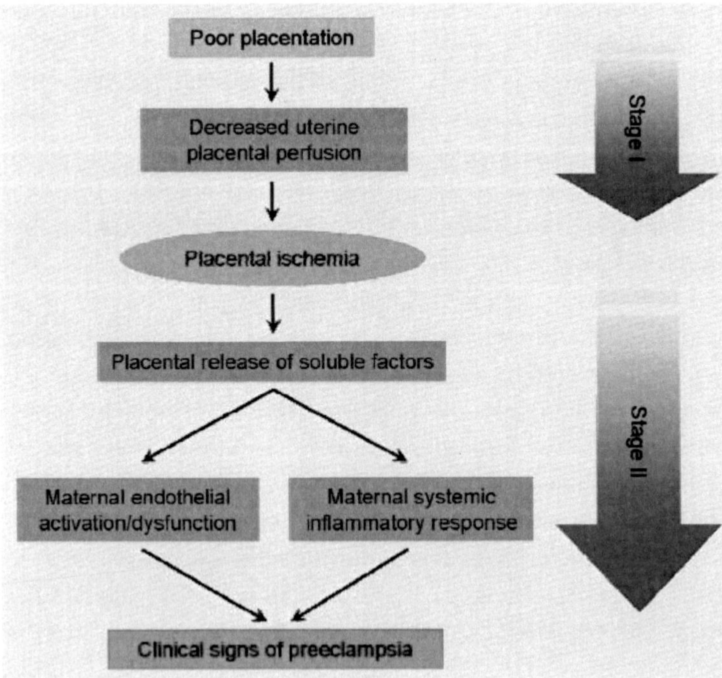

Figure 2. The two-stage model for preeclampsia.

Preeclampsia is a multisystem disorder generally appearing after the 20th week of gestation characterized by hypertension, proteinuria, vascular abnormalities, and possibly intrauterine growth retardation (IUGR) [78-80]. It affects approximately 3–5% of all pregnancies and considered to be one of the leading causes for maternal mortality and a major contributor to maternal and perinatal morbidity. Nevertheless, the mechanisms responsible for the pathogenesis of preeclampsia are poorly understood. The only effective treatment is delivery of the fetus and placenta, often resulting in serious complications of prematurity for the neonate.

Preeclampsia is currently believed to be a two-stage disease [79,81-82]. The first stage is characterized by shallow cytotrophoblast invasion of maternal spiral arterioles, resulting in placental insufficiency. The hypoxic placenta releases soluble factors into the maternal circulation, which induce systemic endothelial dysfunction. This causes the second stage of the disease: the maternal syndrome. During this stage, hypertension and proteinuria, the clinical signs of preeclampsia, are manifested [83] (Figure 2).

4.1. Circulating Angiotensin in Preeclampsia

The RAS has been implicated in the pathogenesis of preeclampsia [27]. While renin, angiotensinogen, Ang II, and aldosterone are increased in the peripheral blood in normal pregnancy [84], in patients with preeclampsia, plasma renin activity and aldosterone are paradoxically suppressed with relatively higher levels of aldosterone for the given level of renin [85-86], suggesting increased adrenal sensitivity to Ang II. Moreover, normal pregnancy is associated with decreased vascular responsiveness to Ang II [31], and preeclampsia is associated with increased sensitivity to Ang II that may develop before the clinical manifestations of the disease [32]. In addition, recent genetic studies have suggested that elevated expression of maternal Ang in human decidual spiral arteries may promote impaired remodeling of these vessels and reduce utero-placental blood flow, potentially initiating for the cascade preceding preeclampsia [12,57] and IUGR [87].

The increased renal sensitivity to Ang II in preeclampsia may be a result of the reduced utero-placental perfusion, and it may be achieved through reductions in nitric oxide (NO) or prostacyclin synthesis or by enhanced formation of thromboxane. Consistent with this suggestion are studies indicating enhanced vascular responsiveness to Ang II in vessels from animals or humans with preeclampsia [29]. Furthermore, previous studies have found that, unlike normal conditions, the preglomerular vessels of the renal circulation become extremely sensitive to the vasoconstrictor actions of Ang II when the renal synthesis of NO or prostacyclin is reduced or when thromboxane synthesis is elevated [88]. Increased vascular Ang II responsiveness during preeclampsia, however, does not prove that Ang II is an important endogenous mediator of the vasoconstriction or hypertension in experimental models of preeclampsia because increased responsiveness may only reflect low endogenous Ang II formation. Thus, the importance of increased Ang II in the regulation of renal function and blood pressure during preeclampsia remains unclear.

4.2 Placental Angiotensin in Preeclampsia

The capacity of the placenta to produce Ang II seems to be also increased in preeclampsia. Recently, increased ACE expression and activity have been reported in placental tissues as well as in umbilical venous plasma samples from pregnancies complicated with preeclampsia [77]. Previously, it has been shown that the level of Ang II in umbilical venous plasma was higher than that in umbilical arterial plasma in preeclamptic placentas and uncomplicated placentas, and that the level of Ang II in maternal peripheral venous plasma was much higher in preeclampsia than in uncomplicated pregnancies [13,89-90]. The level of Ang II in umbilical venous plasma in preeclampsia was also increased as compared to uncomplicated pregnancy, the steeper gradient was noted between umbilical venous and arterial plasma [77]. These data suggest that ACE activity in preeclamptic placenta would be elevated. On the contrary, Kalenga et al did not find any significant differences in placental ACE and Ang II levels between uncomplicated pregnancies and preeclampsia [14]. This controversy may be explained by differences in the investigation methodology used by each group.

4.3. Role of Angiotensin II Receptors

Recent studies in preeclamptic women have revealed several exciting findings regarding the role that Ang II receptors may play in the pathophysiology of preeclampsia. AT1 receptors were shown to form heterodimers with the bradykinin B2 receptor and results in enhanced Ang II sensitivity [91-92]. Further, the AT1-B2 heterodimers are present in greater abundance in preeclamptic women, suggesting that this heterodimerization may play a part in the long observed increased Ang II sensitivity in preeclampsia [91-92].

Furthermore, increased circulating levels of an agonistic autoantibody to the Ang II type 1 receptor (AT1-AA) were demonstrated in preeclamptic women [93-94]. The AT1-AA appear to be responsible for a variety of effects in several different tissues ranging from increased intracellular Ca_{++} mobilization to monocyte activation and stimulation of interleukin (IL)-6 production from mesangial cells [95-98]. While these findings potentially implicate AT1 as a central mediator of several pathways in preeclampsia, both the specific mechanisms that lead to excess production and the mechanisms whereby AT1-AA increases blood pressure during pregnancy remain unclear. Consequently, this has become an area of intense interest.

The AT2 receptors appear to function as an antagonist of AT1 [99]. Increased responsiveness to Ang II has been demonstrated in the uterine vasculature during AT2 receptor blockade [100]. Moreover, enhanced Ang II reactivity has been observed in the uterine vasculature with decreased expression of AT2 in sheep exhibiting preeclampsia-like syndrome after Ang II infusion [101]. Recently, Judson et al., using immunohistochemical techniques, reported that while in normal patients, the level of AT2 receptors is higher than the level of AT1 receptors in patients with preeclampsia this balance is disrupted and the level of AT1 receptors is higher than the level of AT2 receptors [102]. However, more investigations are needed in order to determine whether the expression of AT2 receptors is altered in preeclampsia.

4.4. Angiotensin and Endothelial Dysfunction

Endothelial dysfunction plays a central role in the pathogenesis of the maternal syndrome in preeclampsia. Dysfunctional endothelial cells produce altered quantities of vasoactive mediators, which lead to a tip in the balance towards vasoconstriction [103]. Multiple interconnected pathways including oxidative stress, cytokine release, and a generalized intra-vascular inflammatory response, were reported to be involved in this process. This culminates in increased endothelial cell permeability, lipid peroxidation [104], platelet activation [105], activation of the coagulation cascade, oxidative stress

[106], and a shift in the balance of vasoactive mediators favoring vasoconstriction.

There is accumulating evidence to indicate that Ang II is also capable of inducing inflammatory response in the vascular wall [107]. Characteristic features of inflammation include changes in vascular permeability, recruitment of leukocytes from the circulation to the interstitial tissue, and tissue repair, which involves cell growth and fibrosis [108]. Ang II has been shown to participate in all these processes [107].

Recently, it has been suggested that Ang II, via AT1 receptors, enhances the production of reactive oxygen species (ROS) through stimulation of nicotinamide adenine dinucleotide phosphate [NAD(P)H] oxidase in the vascular wall [109]. Increased oxidative stress contributes to endothelial dysfunction and to vascular inflammation by stimulating the redox-sensitive transcription factor, nuclear factor-kappa B (NF-κB), and by upregulating adhesion molecules, cytokines, and chemokines [107].

Cytokines are messengers for the regulation of the inflammatory cascade, and tumor necrosis factor-α (TNF-α), IL-1β, IL-6 and IL-8 are the main pro-inflammatory cytokines [110]. It has been reported that plasma levels of TNF-α and IL-1β are increased in preeclampsia, whereas conflicting reports on IL-6 and IL-8 show either no difference or increased concentrations [111-115]. Pro-inflammatory cytokines can induce functional and structural alterations, including oxidative damage or interference with the mechanism of concentration/relaxation leading to alterations in vascular integrity, tone and coagulation [110]. Several lines of evidence support the hypothesis that the ischemic placenta in preeclampsia contributes to endothelial cell activation/dysfunction of the maternal circulation by enhancing the synthesis of cytokines such as TNF-α and IL-6 [116].

TNF-α enhances the formation of number of endothelial cell substances such as endothelin and reduces acetylcholine-induced vasodilatation [116]. It has been shown to directly induce oxidative damage as it destabilizes electron flow in mitochondria, resulting in release of oxidizing free radicals and formation of lipid peroxides. Lipid peroxides and oxygen radicals can damage endothelial cells as they are highly reactive compounds. Recently, Ang II has been shown to stimulate the production of cytokines such as TNF-α and IL-6 via the AT1 receptor [117], whereas Ang II receptor blocking attenuated the Ang II stimulated production of these cytokines [118]. Previously, we have shown that stimulation of normal human perfused placenta with Ang II resulted in increased secretion of TNF-α (Figure 3) [28]. These findings suggest that inflammatory cytokines play an important role in mediating the effect of Ang II on the vascular system. On the other hand, TNF-α and IL-1β were shown to act coordinately to increase AT1 receptor density on non-myocytes in the post-MI heart [119].

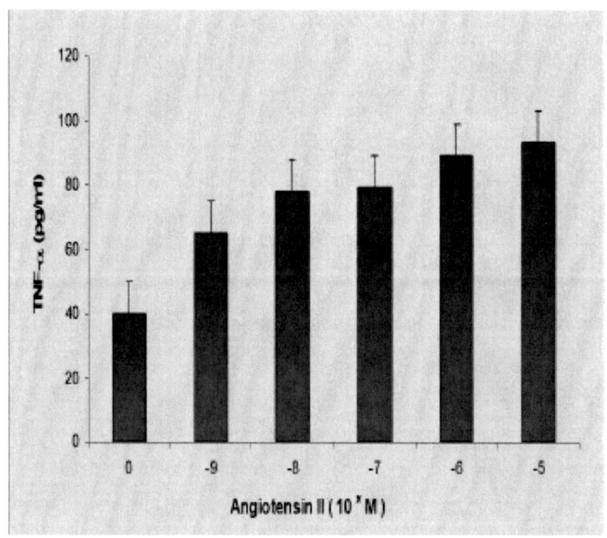

Figure 3. Secretion of TNF-α by normal human placenta before and after Ang II injection ($10^{-9} - 10^{-5}$ M).

5. Magnesium Sulfate and Regulation of Angiotensin II Activity

Magnesium sulfate ($MgSO_4$) is used in pregnancy as prophylaxis and treatment for eclamptic seizures or for preterm labor tocolysis [120]. Magnesium has been shown to reach fetal blood and the amniotic cavity promptly in significant levels following maternal treatment [121-122]. Potential beneficial effects, such as neuro-protection during periods of perinatal hypoxic-ischemia and an association with a decreased risk of cerebral palsy, are being actively studied. Magnesium may improve neonatal outcome through its action on placental vessels. It has been suggested that magnesium may protect against infection-mediated damage by reducing cytokines and bacterial toxin synthesis [123-125].

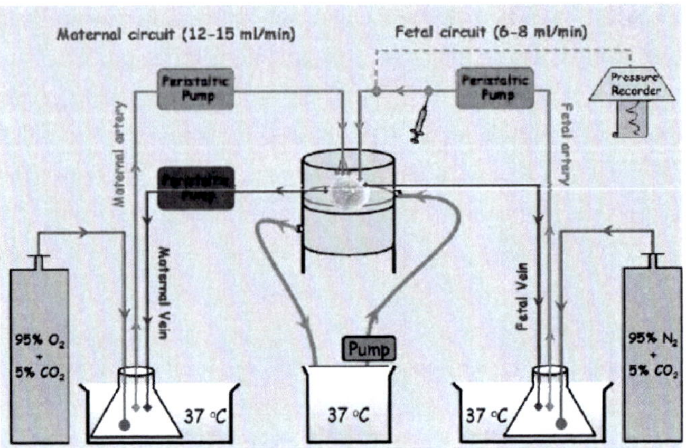

Figure 4. The placental perfusion system as previously described by Schnider and Huch, and modified by Holcberg et al.,.

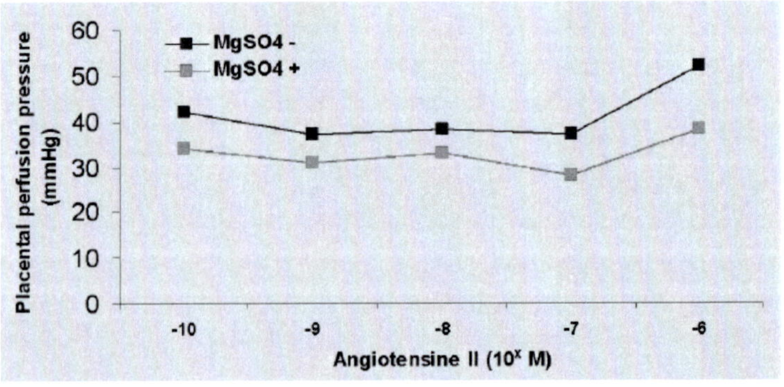

Figure 5. Effect of MgSO4 on Ang II (10-10-10-6M) induced vasoconstriction in perfused human normotensive placenta.

Previously, Kovac et al. reported an increased feto-placental perfusion pressure in placentas from preeclamptic pregnancies, which decreases with exposure to $MgSO_4$ [126]. Moreover, they showed that feto-placental vascular response to Ang II, either in normotensive or in preeclamptic placenta, was not affected by $MgSO_4$. However, recently, using a placental perfusion system previously described by Schneider and Huch [127] and modified by Holcberg et al. (Figure 4) [128], we have shown that $MgSO_4$ selectively attenuates the vasoconstrictor effect of Ang II (Figure 5) and endothelin-1, but not of thromboxane, in the feto-placental vasculature of human normotensive placenta (Figure 5) [128]. The mechanism of action of $MgSO_4$ is thought to be secondary to a competitive inhibition of calcium and its effect on smooth muscle contraction [129].

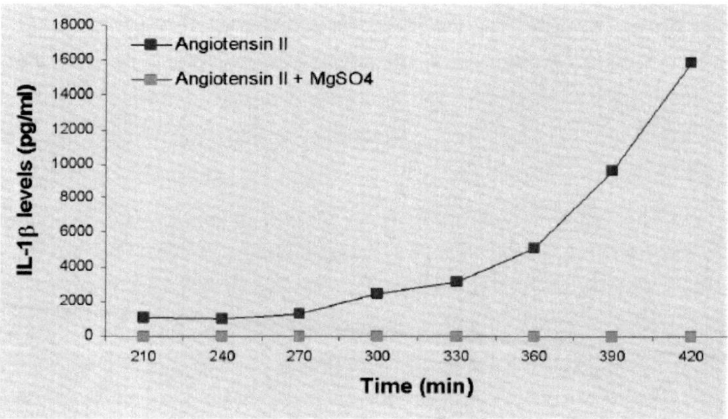

Figure 6. Effect of $MgSO_4$ on Ang II-induced IL-1β secretion by perfused human normotensive placenta.

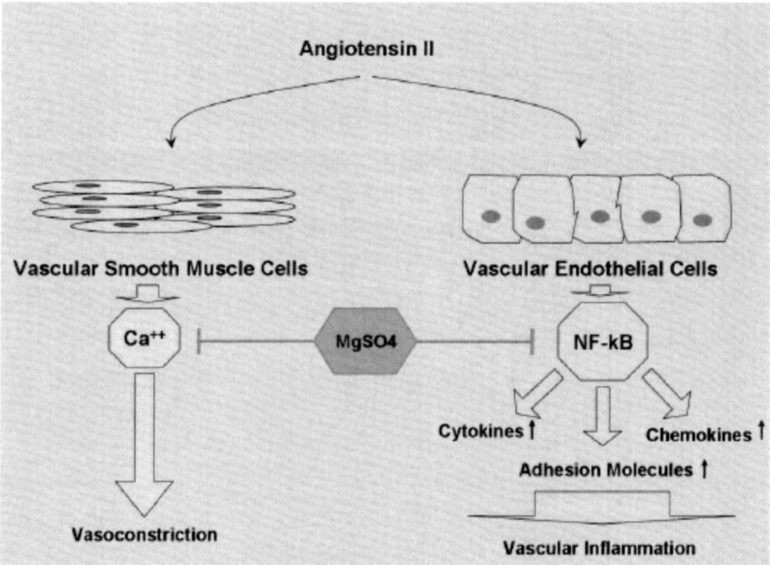

Figure 7. Possible interaction between MgSO4 and Ang II.

Recent findings suggest that $MgSO_4$ may function as an anti-inflammatory agent in certain pathological conditions such as preterm labor

[130], hypertension, vascular disease and stroke [131]. Rochelson et al. suggested that $MgSO_4$ may inhibit endothelial cell activation, as measured by levels of IL-8 and endothelial cell-associated intercellular adhesion molecule-1 (ICAM-1) via NF-κB, and that $MgSO_4$ treatment may function as an anti-inflammatory agent in preterm labor [132]. Since NFκB is one of the main transcription factors mediating Ang II inflammatory response, it is possible to suggest that $MgSO_4$ may be a possible regulator for this response via inhibition of NFκB. Consisting with these suggestion, recently, we have recently shown that $MgSO_4$ attenuates Ang II induced IL-1β secretion by human normotensive perfused placenta (Figure 6) [128]. These data suggest that $MgSO_4$ may be a possible regulator not only of Ang II vasoconstrictor effect on the vascular smooth muscle cells, but also of the inflammatory effect of Ang II on vascular endothelial cells (Figure 7).

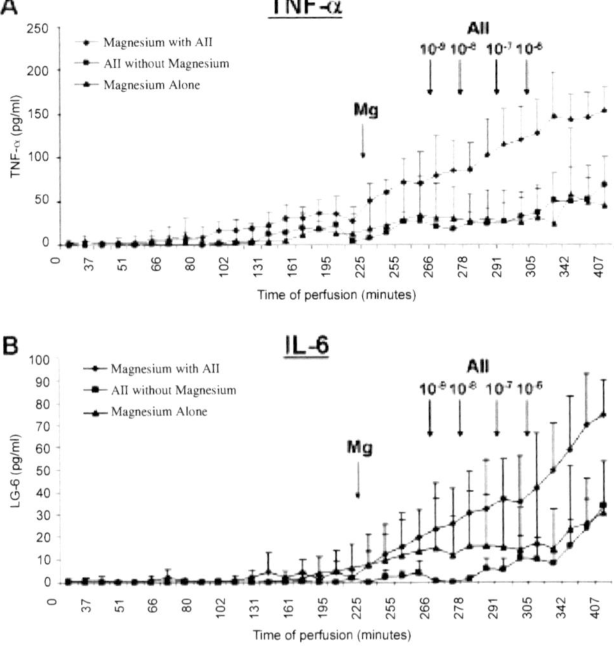

Figure 8. Secretion levels of TNF-α (A) and IL-6 (B) into the maternal compartment of normotensive human term placenta in presence of Ang II alone (four sequential bolus injections into the fetal circuit [10^{-9}-10^{-6} M], at 20 min intervals), $MgSO_4$ alone (6–7mg% in constant infusion into the maternal circuit), and both Ang II and $MgSO_4$ together.

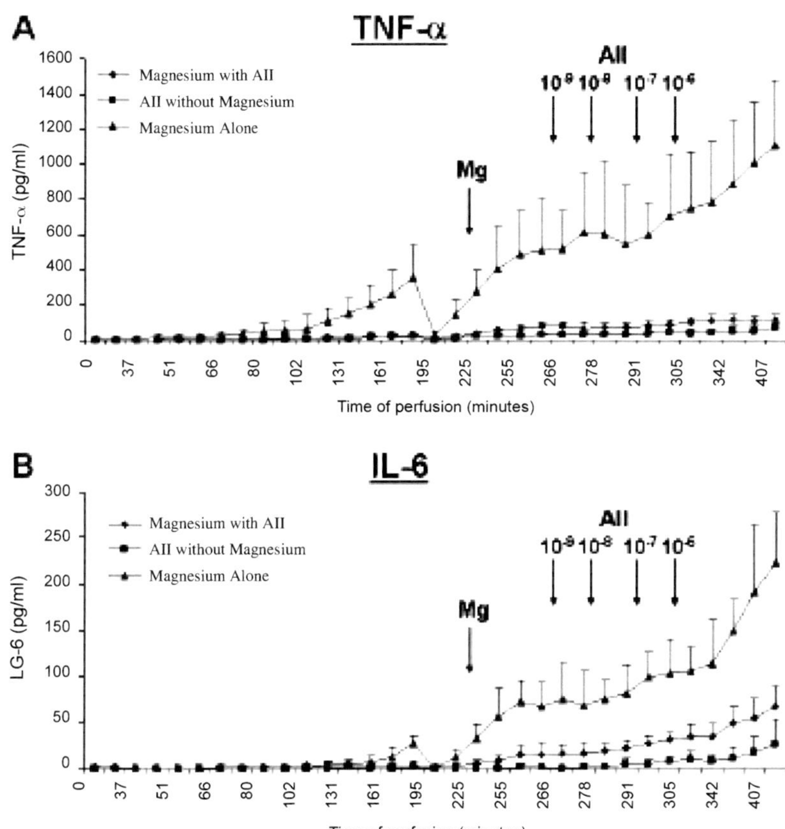

Figure 9. Secretion levels of TNF-α (A) and IL-6 (B) into the fetal compartment of normotensive human term placenta in presence of Ang II alone (four sequential bolus injections into the fetal circuit [10^{-9}-10^{-6} M], at 20 min intervals), $MgSO_4$ alone (6–7mg% in constant infusion into the maternal circuit), and both Ang II and $MgSO_4$ together.

Recently, our group has shown that $MgSO_4$, in addition to its placental vascular vasodilatation effect, may regulate the capacity of human placenta to secrete inflammatory cytokines such as TNF-α and IL-6 [132]. We showed that $MgSO_4$ is capable of increasing TNF-α and IL-6 secretion from the maternal compartment of the human placenta, and that Ang II significantly attenuates this effect (Figure 8A and B). However, in the fetal placental compartment, the interaction of $MgSO_4$ with Ang II leads to a significant increase in TNF-α and IL-6 levels, and $MgSO_4$ alone has no significant effect on TNF-α or IL-6 secretion into the fetal compartment (Figure 9A and B). This may reflect a different response or function of the fetal and maternal compartments of the placenta to these agents. These findings suggest also that $MgSO_4$ may be associated with a significant increase in TNF-α, and IL-6 secretion by the human placenta, and bolus injections of Ang II differently affect secretion of these cytokines into the maternal versus the fetal compartments. The fact that increased levels of TNF-α and IL-6 were secreted into the fetal compartment, after exposure to $MgSO_4$ and Ang II, suggests the possibility of harmful effects of TNF-α to the fetal brain, which may affect late stages of development. Thus, it is possible to suggest that $MgSO_4$, at least partially, could be involved in adverse fetal outcome and the decision for $MgSO_4$ administration during pregnancy should be carefully considered. Further investigation is needed in order to determine this possible interaction between $MgSO_4$ and Ang II in the feto-placental unit.

Conclusion

The conditions for Ang II formation exist and Ang II receptors are present throughout the human utero-placental unit, indicating the presence of a functional local RAS in this organ. Ang II synthesized in the placenta may serve as an autocrine/paracrine modulator of placental function. During normal pregnancy, Ang II levels are elevated although the vascular responsiveness to Ang II appears to be reduced. Ang II is one of the key factors regulating the process of placentation through regulation of trophoblast invasion, angiogenesis and placental vascular development.

Up-regulation of placental RAS might be important for the pathogenesis of some clinical disorders, such as preeclampsia. Increased vascular responsiveness to Ang II, as well as increased placental production of Ang II, were reported in preeclampsia. Moreover, increased AT1 receptor activity was reported in preeclampsia, which may be a result of increased heterodimerization of AT1 with the bradykinin B2 receptor and increased circulating levels of an agonistic autoantibody to the AT1 receptor. Ang II, via AT1 receptor, increases oxidative stress and contributes endothelial dysfunction and to vascular inflammation by stimulating the redox-sensitive transcription factor NF-κB, and by upregulating adhesion molecules, cytokines, and chemokines. $MgSO_4$ may be a possible regulator not only of Ang II vasoconstrictor effect on the vascular smooth muscle cells, but also of the inflammatory effect of Ang II on vascular endothelial cells.

In conclusion, Ang II has significant physiological aspects in reproduction in general, and in placental development and regulation of the utero-placental perfusion in particular. Further studies are still needed in order to assess more accurately the possible interactions between Ang II and $MgSO_4$ in general and the utero-placental unit in particular.

Abbreviations

ACE	angiotensin-converting enzyme;
Ang	angiotensin;
ANP	atrial natriuretic peptide;
AT1	angiotensin II type 1 receptor;
AT1-AA	agonistic autoantibody to the angiotensin II type 1 receptor;
AT2	angiotensin II type 2 receptor;
B2	bradykinin B2 receptor;
BNP	brain natriuretic peptide;
Flt-1	fms-like tyrosine kinase-1;
HIF	hypoxia-inducible factor;
ICAM-1	intercellular adhesion molecule-1;
IL	interleukin;
IUGR	intrauterine growth retardation;
$MgSO_4$	magnesium sulfate;
NAD(P)H	nicotinamide adenine dinucleotide phosphate;
NF-κB	nuclear factor-kappa B;
NO	nitric oxide;
PA	plasminogen activator;
PAH	pregnancy-associated hypertension;
PAI	plasminogen activator inhibitor;
PDGF-β	platelet-derived growth factor-beta;
RAS	renin angiotensin system;
ROS	reactive oxygen species;
TGF-β	transforming growth factor-beta;

TNF-α	tumor necrosis factor-alpha;
VEGF	vascular endothelial growth factor;
VEGF-R	vascular endothelial growth factor receptor.

References

[1] August, P., Lenz, T., Ales, K. L., Druzin, M. L., Edersheim, T. G., Hutson, J. M., Muller, F. B., Laragh, J. H. & Sealey, J. E. (1990). Longitudinal study of the renin-angiotensin-aldosterone system in hypertensive pregnant women: deviations related to the development of superimposed preeclampsia. *Am. J. Obstet. Gynecol.*, *163*, 1612-1621.

[2] Poisner, A. M. (1998). The human placental renin-angiotensin system. *Front. Neuroendocrinol.*, *19*, 232-252.

[3] Hagemann, A., Nielsen, A. H. & Poulsen, K. (1994). *Exp. Clin. Endocrinol.*, *102*, 252-261

[4] Dinh, D. T. (2001). Angiotensin receptors: distribution, signaling and function. *Clin. Science*, *100*, 481-492.

[5] Brede, M. & Hein, L. (2001). Transgenic mouse models of angiotensin receptor subtype function in the cardiovascular system. *Regul. Pept.*, *96*, 125-132.

[6] Ito, M., Oliverio, M. I., Mannon, P. J., Best, C. F., Maeda, N., Smithies, O. & Coffman, T. M. (1995). Regulation of blood pressure by the type 1A angiotensin II receptor gene. *Proc. Natl. Acad. Sci.*, U.S.A., *92*, 3521-3525.

[7] Turner, A. J. & Hooper, N. M. (2002). The angiotensin-converting enzyme gene family: genomics and pharmacology. *Trends Pharmacol. Sci.*, *23*, 177-183.

[8] Meffert, S., Stoll, M., Steckelings, U. M., Bottari, S. P. & Unger, T. (1996). The angiotensin II AT2 receptor inhibits proliferation and promotes differentiation in PC12W cells. *Mol. Cell. Endocrinol.*, *22*, 59-67.

[9] Skinner, S. L., Lumbers, E. R. & Symonds E. M. (1968). Renin concentration in human fetal and maternal tissues. *Am. J. Obstet Gynecol*, *101*, 529-533.

[10] Paul, M., Wagner, J. & Dzau, V. J. (1993). Gene expression of the reninangiotensin system in human tissues. Quantitative analysis by the polymerase chain reaction. *J. Clin. Investig*, *91*, 2058-2064.

[11] Tewksbury, D. A. (1996). Quantification of five forms of high molecular weight angiotensinogen from human placenta. *Am. J. Hypertension*, *9*, 1029-1034.

[12] Morgan, T., Craven, C., Nelson, L., Lalouel, J. M. & Ward, K. (1997). Angiotensinogen T235 expression is elevated in decidual spiral arteries. *J. Clin Investig*, *100*, 1406-1415.

[13] Yagami, H., Kurauchi, O., Murata, Y., Okamoto, T., Mizutani, S. & Tomoda, Y. (1994). Expression of angiotensin-converting enzyme in human placenta and its physiologic role in the fetal circulation. *Obstet. Gynecol*, *84*, 453-457.

[14] Kalenga, M. K., Thomas, K., de Gasparo, M. & de Hertogh, R. (1996). Determination of renin, angiotensin converting enzyme and angiotensin II levels in human placenta, chorion and amnion from women with pregnancy induced hypertension. *Clin. Endocrinol*, *44*, 429-433.

[15] Ito, M., Itakura, A., Ohno, Y., Nomura, M., Senga, T., Nagasaka, T. & Mizutani, S. (2002). Possible activation of the renin–angiotensin system in the feto-placental unit in preeclampsia. *J. Clin. Endocrinol. Metab*, *87*, 1871-1878.

[16] Kalenga, M. K., de Gasparo, M., Thomas, K. & de Hertogh, R. (1996). Review article. Angiotensin II and its different receptor subtypes in placenta and foetal membranes. *Placenta*, *17*, 103-110.

[17] Kalenga, M. K., de Gasparo, M., de Hertogh, R., Whitebread, S., Vankrieken, L. & Thomas, K. (1991). Angiotensin II receptors in the human placenta are type AT1. *Reproduction, Nutrition, Developement*, *31*, 257-267.

[18] Knock, G. A., Sullivan, M. H. F., McCarthy, A., Elder, M. G., Polak, J. M. & Wharton, J. (1994). Angiotensin II (AT1) vascular binding sites in human placentae from normal-term, preeclamptic and growth retarted pregnancies. *J. Pharmacol. Exp. Therapeutics*, *271*, 1007-1015.

[19] Li, X., Shams, M., Zhu, J., Khalig, A., Wilkes, M., Whittle, M., Barnes, N. & Ahmed, A. (1998). Cellular localization of AT1 receptor mRNA and protein in normal placenta and its reduced expression in intrauterine growth restriction. *J. Clin. Investig*, *101*, 442-454.

[20] Sapolsky, A. I. & Woessner, J. F. (1972). Multiple forms of cathepsin D from bovine uterus. *J. Biol. Chem*, *247*, 2069-2076.

[21] Urata, H., Strobel, F. & Ganten, D. (1994). Wide spread tissue distribution of human chymase. *J. Hypertension*, *12*, s17-s22.

[22] Mitzutani, S., Goto, K., Safwat, M., Itakura, A., Kurauchi, O., Kikkawa, F. & Tomoda, Y. (1994). Initiating enzymes of angiotensin II degradation in human placenta and pregnancy serum. *Medical Science Research*, *22*, 537-544.

[23] Hariyama, Y., Itakura, A., Okamura, M., Ito, M., Murata, Y., Nagasaka, T., Nakazato, H. & Mizutani, S. (2000). Placental aminopeptidase A as a possible barrier of angiotensin II between mother and fetus. *Placenta*, *21*, 621-627.

[24] Poston, L. (1997). The control of blood flow to the placenta. *Exp Physiol*, *82*, 377-387.

[25] Boura, A. L., Walters, W. A., Read, M. A. & Leitch, I. M. (1994) Autocoids and control of human placental blood flow. *Clin. Exp. Pharmacol. Physiol*, *21*, 737-748.

[26] Dzau, V. J., Gonzalez, D., Ellison, K., Churchill, S. & Emmett, N. (1987). Characterization of purified rabbit uterine renin: influence of pregnancy on uterine inactive renin. *Endocrinology*, *120*, 358-364.

[27] Nielsen, A. H., Schauser, K. H. & Poulsen, K. (2000). Current topic: the uteroplacental renin-angiotensin system. *Placenta*, *21*, 468-477.

[28] Holcberg, G., Huleihel, M., Sapir, O., Katz, M., Tsadkin, M., Furman, B., Mazor, M. & Myatt, L. (2001). Increased production of tumor necrosis factor-alpha TNF-alpha by IUGR human placentae. *Eur. J. Obstet. Gynecol. Reprod. Biol*, *94*, 69-72.

[29] August, P. & Lindheimer, M. D. (1995). *Hypertension: Pathophysiology of preeclampsia.* (2nd ed). New York, NY: Raven Press.

[30] Shah, D. M. (2005). Role of the renin-angiotensin system in the pathogenesis of preeclampsia. *Am. J. Physiol. Renal. Physiol*, *288*, F614-F625.

[31] Abdul-Karim, R. & Assali, N. (1961). Pressor response to angiotonin in pregnant and nonpregnant women. *Am. J. Obstet. Gynecol.*, *82*, 246-251.

[32] Gant, N. F., Daley, G. L., Chand, S., Whalley, P. J. & MacDonald, P. C. (1973). A study of angiotensin II pressor response throughout primigravid pregnancy. *J. Clin. Invest*, *52*, 2682-2689.

[33] Gant, N. F., Worley, R. J., Everett, R. B. & MacDonald, P. C. (1980). Control of vascular responsiveness during human pregnancy. *Kidney Int*, *18*, 253-258.

[34] Brown, M. A., Gallery, E. D., Ross, M. R. & Esber, R. P. (1988). Sodium excretion in normal and hypertensive pregnancy: a prospective study. *Am. J. Obstet. Gynecol*, *159*, 297-307.

[35] Everett, R. B., Worley, R. J., MacDonald, P. C. & Gant, N. F. (1978). Effect of prostaglandin synthetase inhibitors on pressor response to angiotensin II in human pregnancy. *J. Clin. Endocrinol. Metab*, *46*, 1007-10.

[36] Sanchez-Ramos, L., O'Sullivan, M. J. & Garrido-Calderone, J. (1987). Effect of low-dose aspirin on angiotensin II pressor response in human pregnancy. *Am. J. Obstet. Gynecol*, *156*, 193-4.

[37] Friedman, S. A. (1988). Preeclampsia: A review of the role of prostaglandins. *Obstet. Gynecol*, *71*, 122-37.

[38] Holcberg, G., Kossenjans, W., Brewer, A., Miodovnik, M. & Myatt, L. (1995). The action of two natriuretic peptides (atrial natriuretic peptide and brain natriuretic peptide) in the human placental vasculature. *Am. J. Obstet. Gynecol*, *172*, 71-7.

[39] Dinh, D. T., Frauman, A. G., Johnston, C. I. & Fabiani, M. E. (2001). Angiotensin receptors: distribution, signalling and function. *Clin. Sci*, *100*, 481-492.

[40] Fernandez, L. A., Twickler, J. & Mead, A. (1985). Neovascularization produced by angiotensin II. *J. Lab. Clin. Med*, *105*, 141-145.

[41] Le Noble, F. A. C., Kekking, J. W. M., Van Staaten, H. W. M., Slaaf, D. W. & Struyker Boudier, H. A. (1991). Angiotensin II stimulates angiogenesis in the chorio-allantoic membrane of the chick embryo. *Eur. J. Pharmacol*, *195*, 305-306.

[42] Cooper, A., Robinson, G., Vinson, G., Cheung, W. & Broughton Pipkin, F. (1999). The localization and expression of the renin-angiotensin system in the human placenta throughout pregnancy. *Placenta*, *20*, 467-474.

[43] Li, X., Shams, M., Zhu, J., Khaliq, A., Wilkes, M., Whittle, M., Barnes, N. & Ahmed, A. (1998). Cellular localization of AT1 sub 1 receptor mRNA and protein in normal placenta and its reduced expression in intrauterine growth restriction: angiotensin II stimulates the release of vasorelaxants. *J. Clin. Invest*, *101*, 442-454.

[44] Strickland, S., Reich, E. & Sherman, M. I. (1976). Plasminogen activator in early embryogenesis: enzyme production by trophoblast and parietal endoderm. *Cell*, *9*, 231-240.

[45] Strickland, S. & Beers, W. H. (1976). Studies on the role of plasminogen activator in ovulation. In vitro response of granulosa cells to gonadotropins, cyclic nucleotides, and prostaglandins. *J. Biol. Chem*, *251*, 5694-5702.

[46] Xia, Y., Wen, H. Y. & Kellems, R. E. (2002). Angiotensin II Inhibits Human Trophoblast Invasion through AT1 Receptor Activation. *J. Biol. Chem*, *277*, 24601-8.

[47] Wolf, G. (1998). Angiotensin II is involved in the progression of renal disease: importance of non-hemodynamic mechanisms. *Nephrologie*, *19*, 451-456.

[48] Matsusaka, T., Hymes, J. & Ichikawa, I. (1996). Angiotensin in progressive renal diseases: theory and practice. *J. Am. Soc. Nephrol*, *7*, 2025-2043

[49] Ketteler, M., Noble, N. A. & Border, W. A. (1995). Transforming growth factor-beta and angiotensin II: the missing link from glomerular hyperfiltration to glomerulosclerosis? *Annu. Rev. Physiol*, *57*, 279-295.

[50] Hahn, A. W., Regenass, S., Kern, F., Buhler, F. R. & Resink, T. J. (1993). Expression of soluble and insoluble fibronectin in rat aorta: effects of angiotensin II and endothelin-1. Biochem. *Biophys. Res. Commun*, *192*, 189-197.

[51] Graham, C. & Lala, P. (1991). Mechanism of control of trophoblast invasion in situ. *J. Cell Physiol*, *148*, 228-234.

[52] Graham, C. (1997). Effect of transforming growth factor-beta on the plasminogen activator system in cultured first trimester trophoblast cells. *Placenta*, *18*, 137-143.

[53] Irving, J. & Lala, P. K. (1995). Functional role of cell surface integrins on human trophoblast cell migration: regulation by TGF-beta, IGF-II, and IGFBP-I. *Exp. Cell Res*, *217*, 419-427.

[54] Shaw, K. J., Do, Y. S., Kjos, S., Anderson, P. W., Shinagawa, T., Dubeau, L. & Hsueh, W. A. (1989). Human decidua is a major source of renin. *J Clin Invest*, *83*, 2085-2092.

[55] Morgan, T., Craven, C. & Ward, K. (1998). Human spiral artery renin-angiotensin system. *Hypertension*, *32*, 683-687.

[56] Li, C., Ansari, R., Yu, Z. & Shah, D. (2000). Definitive molecular evidence of renin-angiotensin system in human uterine decidual cells. *Hypertension*, *36*, 159-164.

[57] Morgan, T., Craven, C., Lalouel, J. M. & Ward, K. (1999). Angiotensinogen Thr235 variant is associated with abnormal

physiologic change of the uterine spiral arteries in first-trimester decidua. *Am. J. Obstet. Gynecol*, *180*, 95-102.

[58] Zoumakis, E., Margioris, A. N., Stournaras, C., Dermitzaki, E., Angelakis, E., Makrigiannakis, A., Koumantakis, E. & Gravanis, A. (2000). Corticotrophin-releasing hormone (CRH) interacts with inflammatory prostaglandins and interleukins and affects the decidualization of human endometrial stroma. *Mol. Hum. Reprod*, *6*, 344-351.

[59] Oelkers, W. K. (1996). Effects of estrogens and progestogens on the renin-aldosterone system and blood pressure. *Steroids*, *61*, 166-171.

[60] Shah, D. M., Higuchi, K., Inagami, T. & Osteen, K. G. (1991). Effect of progesterone on renin secretion in endometrial stromal, chorionic trophoblast, and mesenchymal monolayer cultures. *Am. J. Obstet. Gynecol*, *164*, 1145-1150.

[61] Yan, J. S., Guo, L. H., Liu, J. & Wang, H. (1999). Modulation of the secretion of active renin in human decidual cells by progesterone. *Sheng Li Xue Bao*, *51*, 211-218.

[62] Smith, D. L., Law, R. E., Shaw, K. J., Do, Y. S., Hsueh, W. A. & Morris, B. J. (1994). Proximal 6.2 kb of 5'-flanking DNA is insufficient for human renin promoter activity in renin-synthesizing chorio-decidual cells. *Biochim. Biophys. Acta*, *1219*, 465-474.

[63] Sharkey, A. M., Charnock-Jones, D. S., Boocock, C. A., Brown, K. D. & Smith, S. K. (1993). Expression of mRNA for vascular endothelial growth factor in human placenta. *J. Reprod. Fertil*, *99*, 609-615.

[64] Emanueli, C., Salis, M. B., Stacca, T., Pinna, A., Gaspa, L. & Madeddu, P. (2002). Angiotensin AT1 receptor signaling modulates reparative angiogenesis induced by limb ischemia. *Br. J. Pharmacol*, *135*, 87-92.

[65] Munzemaier, D. H. & Greene, A. S. (1996). Opposing actions of antgiotensin II on microvascular growth and arterial blood pressure. *Hypertension*, *27*, 760-5.

[66] Le Noble, F. A., schreurs, N. H., van Straaten, H. W., Slaaf, D. W., Smits, J. F., Rogg, H. & Struijker-Boudier, H. A. (1993). Evidence for a novel angiotensin II receptor involved in angiogenesis in chick embryo chorioallantoic membrane. *Am. J. Physiol*, *264*, R460-5.

[67] Chua, C. C., Hamdy, R. C. & Chua, B. H. (1998). Upregulation of vascular endothelial growth factor by anigiotensin II in rat heart endothelial cells. *Biochem. Biophys. Acta*, *1401*, 187-194.

[68] Williams, B., Baker, A. Q., Gallacher, B. & Lodwick, D. (1995). Angiotensin II increases vascular permeability factor gene expression by human vascular smooth muscle cells. *Hypertension*, *25*, 913-7.

[69] Page, E. L., Robitaille, G. A., Poussegur, J. & Richard, D. E. (2002). Induction of hypoxiainducible factor-1a by transcriptional and translational mechanisms. *J. Biol. Chem*, *277*, 48403-9.

[70] Otani, A., Takagi, H., Suzuma, K. & Honda, Y. (1998). Angiotensin II potentiates vascular endothelial growth factor-induced angiogenic activity in retinal microcapillary endothelial cells. *Circ Res*, *82*, 619-28.

[71] Amaral, S. L., Linderman, J. R., Morse, M. M. & Greene, A. S. (2001). Angiogenesis induced by electrical stimulation is mediated by angiotensin II and VEGF. *Microcirculation*, *8*, 57-67.

[72] Stoll, M., Steckelings, U. M., Paul, M., Bottari, S. P., Metzger, R. & Unger, T. (1995). The angiotensin AT2-receptor mediates inhibition of cell proliferation in coronary endothelial cells. *J. Clin. Invest*, *95*, 651-7.

[73] Benndorf, R., Böger, R. H., Ergün, S., Steenpass, A. & Wieland, T. (2003). Angiotensin II type 2 receptor inhibits vascular endothelial growth factor-induced migration and in vitro tube formation of human endothelial cells. *Circ. Res*, *93*, 438-47.

[74] Clark, D. E., Smith, S. K., He, Y., Day, K. A., Licence, D. R., Corps, A. N., Lammoglia, R. & Charnock-Jones, D. S. (1998). A vascular endothelial growth factor antagonist is produced by the human placenta and released into the maternal circulation. *Biol. Reprod*, *59*, 1540-1548.

[75] Brar, H. S., Kjos, S. L., Dougherty, W., Do, Y. S., Tam, H. B. & Hsueh, W. A. (1987). Increased fetoplacental active renin production in pregnancy-induced hypertension. *Am. J. Obstet. Gynecol*, *157*, 363-367

[76] Leung, P. S., Tsai, S. J., Wallukat, G., Leung, T. N. & Lau, T. K. (2001). The upregulation of angiotensin II receptor AT1 in human preeclamptic placenta. *Mol. Cell Endocrinol*, *184*, 95-102.

[77] Ito, M., Itakura, A., Ohno, Y., Nomura, M., Senga, T., Nagasaka, T. & Mizutani, S. (2002). Possible activation of the renin-angiotensin system in the feto-placental unit in preeclampsia. *J. Clin. Endocrinol. Metab*, *87*, 1871-1878.

[78] Redman, C. W. & Sargent, I. L. (2005). Latest advances in understanding preeclampsia. *Science*, *308*, 1592-1594.

[79] Roberts, J. M. (2000). Preeclampsia: what we know and what we do not know. *Semin Perinatol*, *24*, 24-28.

[80] Granger, J. P., Alexander, B. T., Llinas, M. T., Bennett, W. A. & Khalil, R. A. (2001). Pathophysiology of hypertension during preeclampsia linking placental ischemia with endothelial dysfunction. *Hypertension, 38*, 718-722.

[81] Roberts, J. M. & Cooper, D. W. (2001). Pathogenesis and genetics of pre-eclampsia. *Lancet, 357*, 53-56.

[82] Roberts, J. M. (1998). Endothelial dysfunction in preeclampsia. Semin. Reprod. *Endocrinol, 16*, 5-15.

[83] Ferris, T. F. (1991). Pregnancy, preeclampsia, and the endothelial cell. *N. Engl. J. Med, 325*, 1439-1440.

[84] Skinner, S. L., Lumbers, E. R. & Symonds, E. M. (1972). Analysis of changes in the renin-angiotensin system during pregnancy. *Clin. Sci, 42*, 479-488.

[85] Brown, M. A., Zammit, V. C., Mitar, D. A. & Whitworth, J. A. (1992). Renin-aldosterone relationships in pregnancy-induced hypertension. *Am. J. Hypertens, 5*, 366-371.

[86] Symonds, E. M., Broughton Pipkin, F. & Craven, D. J. (1975). Changes in the renin-angiotensin system in primigravidae with hypertensive disease of pregnancy. *Br. J. Obstet. Gynaecol, 82*, 643-650.

[87] Zhang, X. Q., Varner, M., Dizon-Townson, D., Song, F. & Ward, K. (2003). A molecular variant of angiotensinogen is associated with idiopathic intrauterine growth restriction. *Obstet. Gynecol, 101*, 237-242.

[88] Granger, J. P. & Alexander, B. T. (2000). Abnormal pressure natriuresis in hypertension: Role of nitric oxide. *Acta Physiologica Scandinavia, 168*, 161-168.

[89] Broughton Pipkin, F. & Symonds, E. M. (1977). Factors affecting factor angiotensin II concentrations in the human infant at birth. *Clin. Sci. Mol. Med, 52*, 449-456.

[90] Symonds, E. M. (1979). The placental and the renin-angiotensin system. *J. Reprod. Med, 23*, 129-133.

[91] AbdAlla, S., Lother, H., el Massiery, A. & Quitterer, U. (2001). Increased AT(1) receptor heterodimers in preeclampsia mediate enhanced angiotensin II responsiveness. *Nat. Med*, *7*, 1003-1009.

[92] AbdAlla, S., Lother, H. & Quitterer, U. (2000). AT1-receptor heterodimers show enhanced G-protein activation and altered receptor sequestration. *Nature, 407*, 94- 98.

[93] Wallukat, G., Homuth, V., Fischer, T., Lindschau, C., Horstkamp, B., Jupner, A., Baur, E., Nissen, E., Vetter, K., Neichel, D., Dudenhausen, J. W., Haller, H. & Luft, F. C. (1999). Patients with preeclampsia develop agonistic autoantibodies against the angiotensin AT1 receptor. *J. Clin. Invest*, *103*, 945-952.

[94] Wallukat, G., Neichel, D., Nissen, E., Homuth, V. & Luft, F. C. Agonistic autoantibodies directed against the angiotensin II AT1 receptor in patients with preeclampsia. Can. *J. Physiol. Pharmacol*, *81*, 79-83.

[95] Bobst, S. M., Day, M. C., Gilstrap, L. C., III, Xia, Y. & Kellems, R. E. (2005). Maternal autoantibodies from preeclamptic patients activate angiotensin receptors on human mesangial cells and induce interleukin-6 and plasminogen activator inhibitor-1 secretion. *Am. J. Hypertens*, *18*, 330-336.

[96] Stepan, H., Faber, R., Wessel, N., Wallukat, G., Schultheiss, H. P. & Walther, T. (2006). Relation between Circulating Angiotensin II Type 1 Receptor Agonistic Autoantibodies and Soluble fms-Like Tyrosine Kinase 1 in the Pathogenesis of Preeclampsia. *J. Clin. Endocrinol. Metab*, *91*, 2424-2427.

[97] Walther, T., Wallukat, G., Jank, A., Bartel, S., Schultheiss, H. P., Faber, R. & Stepan, H. (2005). Angiotensin II Type 1 Receptor Agonistic Antibodies Reflect Fundamental Alterations in the Uteroplacental Vasculature. *Hypertension*, *46*, 1275-1279.

[98] Xia, Y., Wen, H., Bobst, S., Day, M. C. & Kellems, R. E. (2003). Maternal autoantibodies from preeclamptic patients activate angiotensin receptors on human trophoblast cells. *J. Soc. Gynecol. Investig*, *10*, 82-93.

[99] AbdAlla, S., Lother, H., Abdel-tawab, A. M. & Quitterer, U. (2001). The angiotensin II AT2 receptor is an AT1 receptor antagonist. *J. Biol. Chem*, *276*, 39721-39726.

[100] McMullen, J. R., Gibson, K. J., Lumbers, E. R., Burrell, J. H. & Wu, J. (1999). Interactions between AT1 and AT2 receptors in uterine arteries from pregnant ewes. *Eur. J. Pharmacol*, *378*, 195-202.

[101] McMullen, J. R., Gibson, K. J., Lumbers, E. R. & Burrell, J. H. (2001). Selective down-regulation of AT2 receptors in uterine arteries from pregnant ewes given 24-h intravenous infusions of angiotensin II. *Regul Pept*, *99*, 119-129.

[102] Judson, J. P., Nadarajah, V. D., Bong, Y. C., Subramaniam, K. & Sivalingam, N. (2006). A preliminary finding: immunohistochemical localisation and distribution of placental angiotensin II receptor subtypes in normal and preeclamptic pregnancies. *Med. J. Malaysia*, *61*, 173-80.

[103] Baumwell, S. & Karumanchi, S. A. (2007). Pre-eclampsia: clinical manifestations and molecular mechanisms. *Nephron Clin. Pract*, *106*, c72-81.

[104] Hubel, C. A., McLaughlin, M. K., Evans, R. W., Hauth, B. A., Sims, C. J. & Roberts, J. M. (1996). Fasting serum triglycerides, free fatty acids, and malondialdehyde are increased in preeclampsia, are positively correlated, and decrease within 48 hours post partum. *Am. J. Obstet Gynecol.*, *174*, 975-982.

[105] Kolben, M., Lopens, A., Blaser, J., Huber, A., Frank, M., Wilhelm, O., Wilhelm, S., Schneider, K. T., Ulm, K., Tschesche, H., et al. (1995). Measuring the concentration of various plasma and placenta extract proteolytic and vascular factors in pregnant patients with HELLP syndrome, pre-/eclampsia and highly pathologic Doppler flow values. *Gynaekol Geburtsh Rundsch*, *35(suppl 1)*, 126-131.

[106] Davidge, S. T. (1998). Oxidative stress and altered endothelial cell function in preeclampsia. *Semin. Reprod. Endocrinol*, *16*, 65-73.

[107] Cheng, Z. J., Vapaatalo, H. & Mervaala, E. (2005). Angiotensin II and vascular inflammation. *Med. Sci. Monit*, *11*, RA194-205.

[108] Touyz, R. M. (2005). Molecular and cellular mechanisms in vascular injury in hypertension: role of angiotensin II. *Curr. Opin. Nephrol. Hypertens*, *14*, 125-131.

[109] Dandona, P., Kumar, V., Aljada, A., Ghanim, H., Syed, T., Hofmayer, D., Mohanty, P., Tripathy, D. & Garg, R. (2003). Angiotensin II receptor blocker valsartan suppresses reactive oxygen species generation in leukocytes, nuclear factor-kappa B, in mononuclear cells of normal subjects: evidence of an antiinflammatory action. *J. Clin .Endocrino. Metab*, *88*, 4496-501

[110] Luppi, P. & Deloia, J. A. (2006). Monocytes of preeclamptic women spontaneously synthesize pro-inflammatory cytokines, *Clin. Immunol.*, *118*, 268-275.

[111] Williams, M. A., Farrand, A., Mittendorf, R., Sorensen, T. K., Zingheim, R. W., O'Reilly, G. C., King, I. B., Zebelman, A. M. & Luthy, D. A. (1999). Maternal second trimester serum tumor necrosis

factor-alpha-soluble receptor p55 (sTNFp55) and subsequent risk of preeclampsia. *Am. J. Epidemiol*, *149*, 323-9.

[112] Kupferminc, M. J., Peaceman, A. M., Wigton, T. R., Tamura, R. K., Rehnberg, K. A. & Socol, M. L. (1994). Immunoreactive tumor necrosis factor-alpha is elevated in maternal plasma but undetected in amniotic fluid in the second trimester. *Am. J. Obstet. Gynecol*, *171(4)*, 976-9.

[113] Greer, I. A., Lyall, F., Perera, T., Boswell, F. & Macara, L. M. (1994). Increased concentrations of cytokines interleukin-6 and interleukin-1 receptor antagonist in plasma of women with preeclampsia: a mechanism for endothelial dysfunction? *Obstet. Gynecol.*, *84(6)*, 937-40.

[114] Al-Othman, S., Omu, A. E., Diejomaoh, F. M., Al-Yatama, M. & Al-Qattan, F. (2001). Differential levels of interleukin 6 in maternal and cord sera and placenta in women with pre-eclampsia. *Gynecol. Obstet. Invest*, *52*, 60-65.

[115] Conrad, K. P., Miles, T. M. & Benyo, D. F. (1998). Circulating levels of immunoreactive cytokines in women with preeclampsia. *Am. J. Reprod. Immunol*, *40*, 102-111.

[116] Conrad, K. P. & Benyo, D. F. (1997). Placental cytokines and the pathogenesis of preeclampsia. *Am J Reprod Immun.*, *37*, 240 -249.

[117] Brasier, A. R. & Recinos, A. 3rd & Eledrisi, M. S. Vascular inflammation and the renin-angiotensin system. *Arterioscler Thromb Vasc Biol*, *22*, 1257-66.

[118] Manabe, S., Okura, T., Watanabe, S., Fukuoka, T. & Higaki, J. (2005). Effects of angiotensin II receptor blockade with valsartan on pro-inflammatory cytokines in patients with essential hypertension. *J. Cardiovasc. Pharmacol*, *46*, 735-9.

[119] Gurantz, D., Cowling, R. T., Varki, N., Frikovsky, E., Moore, C. D. & Greenberg, B. H. (2005). IL-1beta and TNF-alpha upregulate angiotensin II type 1 (AT1) receptors on cardiac fibroblasts and are associated with increased AT1 density in the post-MI heart. *J. Mol. Cell Cardiol*, *38*, 505-15.

[120] Pritchard, J. A. (1979). The use of magnesium sulfate in preeclampsia-eclampsia. *J. Reprod. Med*, *23*, 107-114.

[121] Hankins, G. D., Hammond, T. L. & Yeomans, E. R. (1991). Amniotic cavity accumulation of magnesium with prolonged magnesium sulfate tocolysis. *J. Reprod. Med*, *36*, 446-449.

[122] Hallak, M., Berry, S. M., Madincea, F., Romero, R., Evans, M. I. & Cotton, D. B. (1993). Fetal serum and amniotic fluid magnesium concentrations with maternal treatment. *Obstetr. Gynecol*, *81*, 185-188.

[123] Lipsitz, P. J. & English, I. C. (1967). Hypermagnesemia in the newborn infant. *Pediatrics*, *40*, 856-862.

[124] Nelson, K. B. & Grether, J. K. (1995). Can magnesium sulfate reduce the risk of cerebral palsy in very low birthweight infants? *Pediatrics*, *95*, 263-269.

[125] Hauth, J. C., Goldenberg, R. L., Nelson, K. G., et al. (1995). Reduction of cerebral palsy with maternal magnesium sulfate treatment in newborns weighing 500-1000 g. *Am. J. Obstetr. Gynecol*, *172*, *419*, Abstract #581.

[126] Kovac, C. M., Howard, B. C., Pierce, B. T., Hoeldtke, N. J., Calhoun, B. C. & Napolitano, P. G. (2003). Fetoplacental vascular tone is modified by magnesium sulfate in the preeclamptic ex vivo human placental cotyledon. *Am. J. Obstet. Gynecol*, *189*, 839-42.

[127] Schneider, H. & Huch, A. (1985). Dual in vitro perfusion of an isolated lobe of human placenta: method and instrumentation. *Contrib. Gynecol. Obstetr.*, *13*, 40-47.

[128] Holcberg, G., Sapir, O., Hallak, M., Alaa, A., Shorok, H. Y., David, Y., Katz, M. & Huleihel, M. (2004). Selective vasodilator effect of magnesium sulfate in human placenta. *Am. J. Reprod. Immunol*, *51*, 192-7.

[129] Lewis, D. F. (2005). Magnesium sulfate: the first-line tocolytic. *Obstet. Gynecol. Clin. North Am.*, *32*, 485-500.

[130] Rochelson, B., Dowling, O., Schwartz, N. & Metz, C. N. (2007). Magnesium sulfate suppresses inflammatory responses by human umbilical vein endothelial cells (HuVECs) through the NFkappaB pathway. *J. Reprod. Immunol.*, *73*, 101-7.

[131] Altura, B. M., Kostellow, A. B., Zhang, A., Li, W., Morrill, G. A., Gupta, R. K. & Altura, B. T. (2003). Expression of the nuclear factor-kappaB and proto-oncogenes c-fos and c-jun are induced by low extracellular Mg2+ in aortic and cerebral vascular smooth muscle cells: possible links to hypertension, atherogenesis, and stroke. *Am. J. Hypertens.*, *16*, 701-7.

[132] Holcberg, G., Amash, A., Sapir, O., Hallak, M., Sheiner, E., Ducler, D., Katz, M. & Huleihel, M. (2006). Different effects of magnesium sulfate and angiotensin II on the capacity of the fetal and maternal

compartments of normal human placenta to secrete TNF-alpha and IL-6. *J. Reprod. Immunol.*, *69*, 115-25.

In: Human Placenta: Structure and Development... ISBN: 978-1-60876-457-0
Editors: E. Berven, et al. pp. 213-229 © 2010 Nova Science Publishers, Inc.

Chapter IX

Fusogenic Syncytin-1 and Transcription Factor Glial Cells Missing-A: Presumed Regulators in Human Placental Physiology and Pathophysiology

Christina Wich[1], Said Hashemolhosseini[2] and Ina Knerr[*3]

[1]Department of Medicine, University of Erlangen-Nuremberg, Erlangen, Germany.

[2]Institute of Biochemistry, University of Erlangen-Nuremberg, Germany.

[3]Children's and Adolescents' Hospital, University of Erlangen-Nuremberg, Erlangen, Germany.

Abstract

The differentiation process and cell-cell fusion of human trophoblasts in the human placenta are controlled by a variety of regulatory genes and key molecules. In this article, we focus on the fusogenic glycoprotein syncytin-1, which originally derived from the human endogenous retrovirus HERV-W. In addition, we look at its transcription factor GCMa (glial cells missing-a or Gcm1).

---

[*] Corresponding author: Email: ina.knerr@uk-erlangen.de, Tel: ++49 9131 85-33118; Fax: ++49 9131 85-33113.

We propose that GCMa-driven syncytin-1 expression is a key mechanism for syncytiotrophoblast formation in the human placenta. Besides the physiological significance of syncytin-1 and GCMa, we discuss their pathophysiological role in pre-eclampsia and intrauterine growth restriction (IUGR). In addition, we focus on the effects of hypoxia on the expression of syncytin-1 and GCMa in trophoblastic cells because changing oxygen availability contributes to abnormal placental development. Basically, any alteration of the cAMP signaling cascade involving protein kinase A (PKA), GCMa and syncytin-1 can be considered a major risk factor for diminished trophoblast differentiation and impaired syncytiotrophoblast formation, followed by placental dysfunction, for example, in the course of hypoxia. Furthermore, hypoxia-related down-regulation of syncytin-1 can, to a great extent, be compensated by stimulating the cAMP-driven PKA pathway. Considering that pre-eclampsia is unique to humans and that syncytin-1 is derived from the HERV-W family exclusively found in humans and in higher primates, syncytin-1 is an interesting candidate for research into human placental physiology and altered placental function.

Similarly, we describe a putative mode of action at the cellular level. Using a cell culture model of syncytin-1 overexpressing cells it has been shown that syncytin-1 is capable of anti-apoptotic functions. A lower apoptotic response, such as a lower level of caspase 3 along with higher amounts of anti-apoptotic Bcl-2 have been found in syncytin-1 transfected cells compared with controls.

In conclusion, we propose that fusogenic syncytin-1 may function as an anti-apoptotic glycoprotein during cell-cell fusion processes. Conversely, alterations in the syncytin-1/GCMa system may, in certain circumstances, be followed by placental disturbances and disorders of pregnancy such as pre-eclampsia and IUGR.

Introduction

The human placenta is essential for the intrauterine development of the fetus, but is also involved in programming health in later life (Plagemann et al., 2008). This organ is an interesting tool for studying the fundamental processes of cell differentiation and cell-cell fusion controlled by a variety of regulatory genes and key molecules.

In this review we focus on the fusogenic glycoprotein syncytin-1, which originally derived from the human endogenous retrovirus HERV-W, and its transcription factor GCMa (glial cells missing-a or Gcm1). We discuss their putative role in normal human placentogenesis and in hypertensive disorders of pregnancy such as pre-eclampsia and intrauterine growth restriction (IUGR).

Syncytin-1, A Placental Fusogenic Protein

Syncytin-1, the envelope (Env) protein of the human endogenous retrovirus HERV-W was first described in 2000 (Mi et al., 2000, Blond et al. 2000). It has been shown that this endogenous retroviral particle was involved in the formation of cell syncytia, which is an essential mechanism during placentogenesis. The application of antisense oligonucleotides against syncytin-1 was followed by an inhibition of cell-cell fusion and impaired trophoblast cell differentiation (Frendo et al., 2003b). Accordingly, fusogenic syncytin-1 is considered to be a key player in normal human placentogenesis (Frendo et al., 2003b, Knerr et al., 2004). The syncytin-1 gene maps to chromosome 7q21-7q22 (OMIM 604659). More recently, other HERV families have been described, and the Env protein of one of them, HERV-FRD, was named syncytin-2 (Blaise et al. 2003). However, the physiological role of syncytin-2 is, as yet, unknown.

Syncytin-1 is predominantly found in the syncytiotrophoblast of the human placenta. Its localization seems to vary during pregnancy. In detail, syncytin-1 is expressed at the apical membrane site during the 1st trimenon and in term placental tissue, and at the basal site of the syncytiotrophoblast in the 2nd and 3rd trimenon placenta (Frendo et al., 2003b, Blond et al., 2000, Lee et al. 2001).

The syncytiotrophoblast forms a selective maternal-fetal barrier in the human placenta and this essential cell layer is formed by the cell-cell fusion of villous cytotrophoblasts. Moreover, it provides the transport interface between the mother and fetus regulating oxygen exchange, metabolic supply and endocrine functions such as the production of steroid hormones, human chorionic gonadotropin (hCG) and human placental lactogen (hPL) (Bischof et al., 2005).

In principle, fusion processes between trophoblastic cells can be stimulated by endothelial growth factor (EGF), hCG, estrogen and dexamethason. Moreover, an upregulation of trophoblastic cell function occurs via the cyclic adenosine monophosphate (cAMP), cAMP-dependent protein kinase A (PKA) pathway (Kudo et al., 2002; Knerr et al., 2005). The placental differentiation markers hCG and hPL are increased following syncytial differentiation, and syncytin-1 mRNA and glycoprotein expression are colinear with cytotrophoblast differentiation and hCG expression (Frendo et al., 2003b). Following stimulation with cAMP agonists or the adenylate cyclase activator forskolin, human trophoblasts exhibit a rapid increase of syncytin-1 transcripts within the first 24h of culture along with its transcription factor GCMa (Figure 1). In addition, syncytin-1 transcript levels in placental villi specimens are positively correlated with gestational age (Knerr et al., 2004).

The syncytiotrophoblast forms a selective maternal-fetal barrier in the human placenta and this essential cell layer is formed by the cell-cell fusion of villous cytotrophoblasts. Moreover, it provides the transport interface between the mother and fetus regulating oxygen exchange, metabolic supply and endocrine functions such as the production of steroid hormones, human chorionic gonadotropin (hCG) and human placental lactogen (hPL) (Bischof et al., 2005).

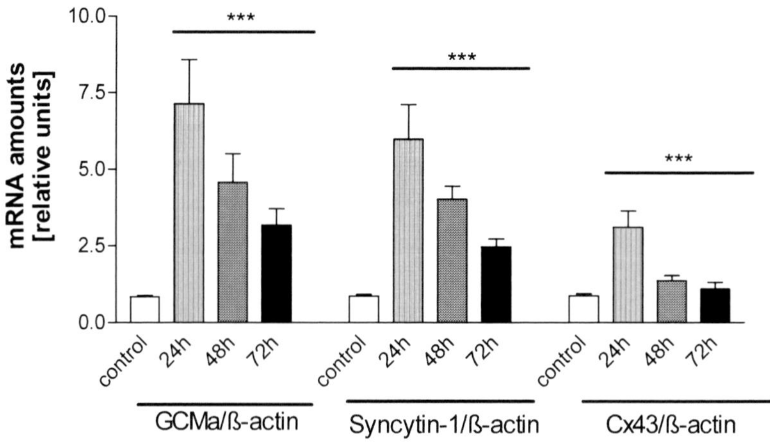

Figure 1. Gene expression of GCMa, syncytin-1 and connexin43 (Cx43) normalized to ß-actin in primary term human trophoblasts after incubation at normoxia (21%O_2) with 100 µM forskolin for different incubation periods (24h, 48h and 72h). $p<0.001$ (***) vs. unstimulated controls. Methodological details are reported elsewhere (Knerr et al., 2005). Following an early increase, we observed a progressive decrease of syncytin-1 and GCMa transcripts after 48h of cell culture, indicative of a regulatory limitation of the fusion process. Peak levels of Cx43 mRNA were found after 24h of culture which is related to an initiation of syncytialisation and activation of gap junctions.

In principle, fusion processes between trophoblastic cells can be stimulated by endothelial growth factor (EGF), hCG, estrogen and dexamethason. Moreover, an upregulation of trophoblastic cell function occurs via the cyclic adenosine monophosphate (cAMP), cAMP-dependent protein kinase A (PKA) pathway (Kudo et al., 2002; Knerr et al., 2005). The placental differentiation markers hCG and hPL are increased following syncytial differentiation, and syncytin-1 mRNA and glycoprotein expression are colinear with cytotrophoblast differentiation and hCG expression (Frendo et al., 2003b). Following stimulation with cAMP agonists or the adenylate cyclase activator forskolin, human trophoblasts exhibit a rapid increase of syncytin-1 transcripts within the first 24h of culture along with its transcription factor GCMa (Figure 1).

In addition, syncytin-1 transcript levels in placental villi specimens are positively correlated with gestational age (Knerr et al., 2004).

Transcription Factor GCMa (Glial Cells Missing A)

Glial cells missing a (GCMa), discovered in Drosophila, is a member of a transcription factor family characterized by a zinc-containing DNA binding domain at its aminoterminus (Cohen et al., 2003). Two different family members are known in mammals: GCMa is found in syncytiotrophoblast, thymus, kidneys and astrocytes, GCMb in parathyroid tissue (Hashemolhosseini and Wegner, 2004).

Two GCMa binding sites have been identified in the syncytin-1 promoter region (Janatpour et al., 1999) which supports the assumption that syncytin-1 is a target gene of GCMa (Prudhomme et al., 2004, Yu et al., 2002). We have described in detail the cAMP-driven PKA-dependent/GCMa/syncytin-1 signaling pathway (Knerr et al., 2005; Figure 2). Recently, we reported that the cAMP-PKA pathway activates bZIP-type transcription factors CREB (cAMP response–element binding protein) and OASIS (old astrocyte specifically-induced substance), thereby stimulating GCMa gene transcription (Schubert et al., 2008). Moreover, there are other posttranslational events that modulate GCMa activity, like CBP (CREB binding protein)-mediated acetylation (Chang et al., 2005).

Connexin 43, A Putative Effector Molecule

At the cellular level, syncytialisation requires an up-regulation of cell-cell communication and contact. Cellular interaction is enabled by gap junctions localized in the plasma membrane. They allow the exchange of metabolites and signaling molecules such as Ca^{2+} and cAMP. Gap junctions are constructed of eight membrane proteins called connexins (Cx). Several different Cx families can be found in the placenta. It appears that Cx43 is required for the fusion of cytotrophoblasts to build the syncytiotrophoblast, whereas Cx40 may play a role in the switch from a proliferative to an invasive phenotype of cytotrophoblast (Cronier et al., 2003, Knerr et al., 2005, Malassiné and Cronier, 2005). It has been shown that a stimulation of the cAMP/PKA signaling pathway leads to a CREB / OASIS / GCMa-dependent increased expression of Cx43 and the simultaneous loss of adherence markers such as desmosomal desmoplakin (Douglas et al., 1990; Knerr et al., 2005, Schubert et al., 2008). Direct interaction of Cx43 in cell-cell fusion has been demonstrated using antisense oligonucleotides which was followed by a reduced fusion rate and altered expression of syncytin-1 and hCG (Frendo et al., 2003a). Conversely, higher amounts of GCMa and syncytin mRNA are followed by higher Cx43 expression levels in human trophoblasts (Figure 1).

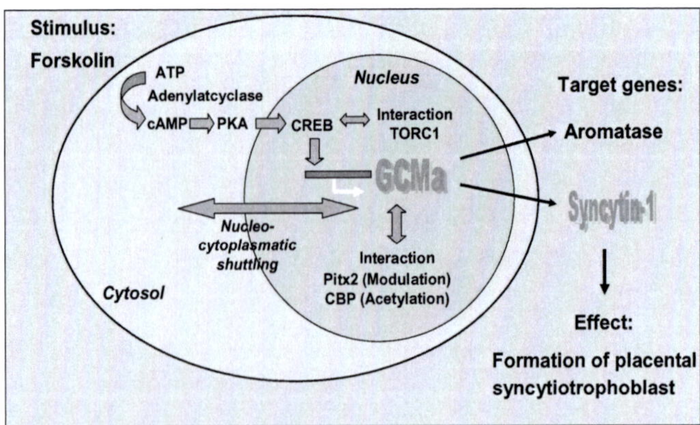

Figure 2. Model demonstrating the known mechanisms of regulation and target genes of syncytin-1 in trophoblastic cells. One of the master regulators of placental cell fusion is the transcription factor GCMa which is regulated at different levels within a network of other transcription factors. The cAMP-driven protein kinase A signaling pathway is fundamental for the up-regulation of GCMa and syncytin-1. Further details are presented elsewhere (Schubert el., 2008).

Human Endogenous Retroviruses (HERVs)

In the 1970s, investigations on baboon placentas using electron microscopy revealed the existence of HERVs. Distinctive particles, having strong similarities to retroviruses, were punched of the syncytiotrophoblast (Ryan et al., 2004, Harris et al., 1998). About 5-8% of the human genome consists of retroviral genome sequences derived from the typical retroviral gene sequence 5'-LTR-gag-pol-env-LTR-3' (Gifford et al., 2003; Medstrand et al., 2002, Bannert et al., 2004). However, during the past million years, open reading frames are rarely kept intact and genetic information has been lost due to mutations. The origin of HERVs is still not clear and there are several different theories. HERVs could be the legacy of ancient germ cell infections by exogenous retroviruses, dating from 60 million years ago to the present (Ryan et al., 2004). In many cases, however, exogenous counterparts could not be identified, or may have disappeared (Loewer et al., 1996).

It seems that HERVs could be involved in various pathologies in humans. HERV elements have been detected in malignancies such as seminoma, chorioncarcinoma, breast cancer, and renal cancer, but a direct activation of oncogenes could not be demonstrated (Gifford et al., 2003; Nelson et al., 2004; Ryan et al., 2004). Moreover, hereditary diseases have been discussed in the context of HERV-related elements, induced mutations and altered gene expression, including neurofibromatosis or Lesch Nyhan syndrome (Ryan et al., 2004). In the cerebrospinal fluid of patients with multiple sclerosis high amounts of HERV-W transcripts have been detected, which could be depressed following successful treatment with interferone ß. Conversely, interferone γ and TNF α activate macrophages which may be followed by an overexpression of HERV-W (Johnston et al., 2001; Taruscio et al., 2004). Therefore, the physiological and pathophysiological role of HERV-W during inflammation is, as yet, unclear.

It is of interest to know that syncytin-1 covers a 25-amino acid sequence (residues 373 to 397) conserved in other retroviral envelope proteins which mediates immunosuppression (Mangeney et al., 2007). This may explain the immune tolerance of cells to HERV. The placenta should protect the fetus against the maternal immune system and resist infection (Muir et al., 2004). Retroviral envelopes could theoretically mediate such functions with receptor interference, and their immunosuppression and fusion properties.

Conversely, dysfunction of the maternal immune system may contribute to an increased release of placental cell detritus into the maternal circulation, systemic inflammatory reaction and, eventually, clinical symptoms such as in pre-eclampsia (Sacks et al., 1998; Bachmayer et al., 2006). It may be that reduced syncytin-1 expression, together with an altered distribution in the syncytiotrophoblast, plays a pathophysiological role, especially through a diminished immunosuppressive effect in the placenta.

Clinical Context: Hypertensive Disorders of Pregnancy

Disorders of placental development may be followed by increased maternal and fetal morbidity, in particular hypertensive disorders of pregnancy such as pre-eclampsia or the HELLP syndrome, and fetal intrauterine growth restriction (IUGR). Pre-eclampsia is defined by the onset of arterial hypertension (blood pressure >140/90mmHg), proteinuria with renal dysfunction (> 300mg protein excretion/24h) and peripheral edema. The HELLP syndrome is characterized by hemolysis, elevated liver enzymes and low platelets.

Disease specific incidences are 6% to 8% for hypertensive disorders in general and 3.9/1000 pregnancies for severe pre-eclampisa, 0.5/1000 for the HELLP syndrome, 0.2/1000 for eclampsia with convulsions (Waterstone et al., 2001, Report of the National High Blood Pressure Education Program Working Group on High Blood Pressure in Pregnancy, 2000). Etiology and pathogenesis of hypertensive disorders of pregnancy are multifactorial and still not completely understood. Essentially, maternal risk factors for endothelial and vascular diseases, such as preexisting arterial hypertension and diabetes mellitus, predispose to these disorders (Al-Muhamid et al., 2003). It is of interest that clinical symptoms occur as late as the 2nd and at 3rd trimenon of pregnancy, while placental alterations start early in placentogenesis. A possible explanation could be that disturbed placentogenesis with reduced syncytiotrophoblast formation may manifest only after placental volume and fetal demands increase.

Histological investigations exhibit poor invasion of cytotrophoblasts in maternal uterine arteries along with disturbed remodelling of spiral arteries. Large intervillous lacunae in the placenta which, under normal conditions, are responsible for adequate blood supply are formed in a defective way, which may result in a chronic hypoxic state (Pijnenborg et al., 1998, Redman and Sargent, 2003). As a consequence, pre-eclampsia can be associated with IUGR. It is of interest to know that comparable processes are not well documented in other species (Redman and Sargent, 2003).

Syncytin and GCMa: Alterations in Pre-Eclampsia and Under-Hypoxia

Syncytin-1 gene expression is reduced in placentas of women with pre-eclampsia or HELLP syndrome (Knerr et al., 2002; Chen et al., 2006). Additionally, altered protein localization in the apex of the syncytiotrophoblast was observed (Lee et al., 2001). Considering that pre-eclampsia is typically associated with local hypoxia, it was of interest to focus on syncytin-1 expression under experimental hypoxia. A decrease of syncytin-1 and GCMa expression could be demonstrated (Knerr et al., 2005, Kudo et al., 2003). Reduced oxygen availability in the placenta may lead to a reduced syncytin-1 gene expression which, in certain circumstances, may be followed by disturbed placentogenesis.

Normal placental cell differentiation of cytotrophoblasts to the syncytiotrophoblast layer is reduced under hypoxia and the proliferative cell phenotype increases (Soleymanlou et al., 2005). Consequently, defective fusion processes occur and can be demonstrated, for example, by a decreased immunocytochemical detection of Cx43 and persistent desmoplakin staining. To a certain extent, stimulation of the cAMP/PKA-pathway can attenuate hypoxia-related effects and facilitate syncytialization (Knerr et al., 2005). The cellular mechanisms include many other elements and need to be further elucidated.

Syncytin Receptor, the Amino Acid Transporter ASCT2

The first known syncytin binding site is a sodium-dependent neutral amino acid transporter at the basal membrane of syncytiotrophoblast, which transports alanine, serine, and cysteine. It is named by the acronym ASCT2 or type D retrovirus receptor, RDR (Sommerfelt et al. 1990; Rasko et al., 1999; Kudo and Boyd, 2002). Syncytin-1 is also capable of binding to the transporter ASCT1 (Marin et al., 2000). The degree of structural homology between ASCT1 and 2 is 57% (Zerangue et al., 1996, Kudo and Boyd, 2002). In transfected CHO cells, intercellular fusion of ASCT1 overexpressing cells was even higher than the fusion rate of ASCT2-transfected cells (Lavilette et al., 2002). In humans, ASCT1 is predominantly found in liver and brain.

During the process of syncytialisation, syncytin-1 mRNA amounts increase in 1st trimenon placental tissue, but ASCT2 receptor expression decreases after the 13th week of gestation which could be interpreted as a limitation of cell-cell fusion (Chen et al., 2006). In placentas of women with pre-eclampsia or HELLP syndrome an almost constant ASCT2 mRNA level could be detected throughout pregnancy (Chen et al., 2006). ASCT2 gene expression is not significantly affected under hypoxic cell culture conditions (Knerr et al., 2003). Moreover, ASCT2 expression is down-regulated after stimulation of trophoblast cell fusion, and not associated with the proliferative status of trophoblasts (Hayward et al., 2007).

Interaction of Syncytin-1 with Apoptosis Elements

Apoptosis, or programmed cell death, is an essential mechanism in early human development and for maintaining tissue homeostasis. Early apoptotic steps and syncytium formation share common mechanisms, such as changes in plasma membrane phospholipid orientation, particularly the phosphatidylserin-flip (Poetgens et al., 2002, Lyden et al., 1993). In trophoblasts, however, cell death seems to be deferred after fusion processes, and the apoptotic cascade initiated in the villous cytotrophoblast, in turn promotes syncytial fusion (Huppertz et al., 1998). Using a cell culture model of syncytin-1 overexpressing cells it has been shown that syncytin-1 is capable of anti-apoptotic functions. A lower apoptotic response has been found in syncytin-1 transfected cells compared with mock transfectants, in particular, a lower level of executioner caspase 3 along with higher amounts of anti-apoptotic Bcl-2 (Knerr et al. 2007).

Excursion: Mouse Placenta

In the mouse placenta, fusogenic Env proteins of retroviral origin have been also detected and labeled, in analogy to syncytin-1 and 2, syncytin-A and B (Dupressoir et al., 2005). There is a high conformity in genomic sequence and protein structure between the human and mouse Env proteins which may be helpful for further studies of normal and abnormal pregnancies (Peng et al., 2007).

Constitutive knockout mice for GCMa show embryonal death at mid gestation. Embryonic malformation was not observed, so an underlying placental pathology was suspected. In detail, GCMa knockouts are unable to develop a functional syncytiotrophoblast layer and as a consequence the embryo can not be supplied by sufficient amounts of nutrients and oxygen (Schreiber et al., 2000). Syncytin-1/A knockout mice are not available.

Conclusion

Formation of the placental syncytiotrophoblast is a complex process. Its success, together with a normal development of fetus and placenta, is regulated by various factors. We propose that syncytin-1, a glycoprotein of endogenous retroviral origin, may exert fusogenic, anti-apoptotic and immune modulatory properties and heretofore unknown influences on the cell membrane which together facilitate cell-cell fusion between trophoblasts. Alterations of this process, such as hypoxic conditions, may eventually lead to disorders of pregnancy such as pre-eclampsia and IUGR.

References

[1] Al-Mulhim, A. A., Abu-Heija, A., Al-Jamma, F. & El-Harith, el-H.A. (2003). Pre-eclampsia: maternal risk factors and perinatal outcome. *Fetal Diagn Ther.*, *18*, 275-80.

[2] Bachmayer, N., Rafik Hamad, R., Liszka, L., Bremme, K. & Sverremark-Ekström, E. (2006). Aberrant uterine natural killer (NK)-cell expression and altered placental and serum levels of the NK-cell

promoting cytokine interleukin-12 in pre-eclampsia. *Am J Reprod Immunol.Am. J. Reprod. Immunol.*, *56*, 292-301.

[3] Bannert, N. & Kurth, R. (2004). Retroelements and the human genome: new perspectives on an old relation. *Proc Natl Acad SciProc. Natl. Acad. Sci.*, USA., *101 Suppl 2*, 14572-9.

[4] Bischof, P. & Irminger-Finger, I. (2005). The human cytotrophoblastic cell, a mononuclear chameleon. *Int J BiochemInt. J. Biochem. Cell Biol.*, *37*, 1-16.

[5] Blaise, S., de Parseval, N., Bénit, L. & Heidmann, T. (2003). Genomewide screening for fusogenic human endogenous retrovirus envelopes identifies syncytin 2, a gene conserved on primate evolution. *Proc Natl Acad SciProc. Natl. Acad. Sci.*, U S A., *100*, 13013-8.

[6] Blond, J. L., Lavillette, D., Cheynet, V., Bouton, O., Oriol, G., Chapel-Fernandes, S., Mandrand, B., Mallet, F. & Cosset, F. L. (2000). An envelope glycoprotein of the human endogenous retrovirus HERV-W is expressed in the human placenta and fuses cells expressing the type D mammalian retrovirus receptor. *J. Virol.*, *74*, 3321-9.

[7] Chang, C. W., Chuang, H. C., Yu, C., Yao, T. P. & Chen, H. (2005). Stimulation of GCMa transcriptional activity by cyclic AMP/protein kinase A signaling is attributed to CBP-mediated acetylation of GCMa. *Mol. Cell Biol.*, *25*, 8401-14.

[8] Chen, C. P., Wang, K. G., Chen, C. Y., Yu, C., Chuang, H. C. & Chen, H. (2006). Altered placental syncytin and its receptor ASCT2 expression in placental development and pre-eclampsia. *BJOG.*, *113*, 152-8.

[9] Cohen, S. X., Moulin, M., Hashemolhosseini, S., Kilian, K., Wegner, M. & Muller, C. W. (2003). Structure of the GCM domain-DNA complex: a DNA-binding domain with a novel fold and mode of target site recognition. *EMBO J.*, *22*, 1835-45.

[10] Cronier, L., Frendo, J. L., Defamie, N., Pidoux, G., Bertin, G., Guibourdenche, J., Pointis, G. & Malassine, A. (2003). Requirement of gap junctional intercellular communication for human villous trophoblast differentiation. *Biol. Reprod.*, *69*, 1472-80.

[11] Douglas, G. C. & King, F. (1990). Differentiation of human trophoblast cells in vitro as revealed by immunocytochemical staining of desmoplakin and nuclei. *J. Cell Sci.*, *96*, 131-141.

[12] Dupressoir, A., Marceau, G., Vernochet, C., Bénit, L., Kanellopoulos, C., Sapin, V. & Heidmann, T. (2005). Syncytin-A and syncytin-B, two fusiogenic placenta-specific murine envelope genes of retroviral origin

conserved in Muridae. *Proc Natl Acad SciProc. Natl. Acad. Sci.*, U S A., *18*, *102*, 725-30.

[13] Frendo, J. L., Cronier, L., Bertin, G., Guibourdenche, J., Vidaud, M., Evain-Brion, D. & Malassine, A. (2003). Involvement of connexin43 in human trophoblast cell fusion and differentiation. *J. Cell Sci.*, *116(Pt 16)*, 3413-21.(a)

[14] Frendo, J. L., Olivier, D., Cheynet, V., Blond, J. L., Bouton, O., Vidaud, M., Rabreau, M., Evain-Brion, D. & Mallet, F. (2003). Direct involvement of HERV-W Env glycoprotein in human trophoblast cell fusion and differentiation. *Mol. Cell Biol.*, *23*, 3566-74.(b)

[15] Gifford, R. & Tristem, M. (2003). The evolution, distribution and diversity of endogenous retroviruses. *Virus Genes.*, *26*, S.291-315.

[16] Harris, J. R. (1998). Placental endogenous retrovirus (ERV): structural, functional, and evolutionary significance. *Bioassays.*, *20*, 307-16.

[17] Hashemolhosseini, S. & Wegner, M. (2004). Impacts of a new transcription factor family: mammalian GCM proteins in health and disease. *J. Cell Biol.*, *166*, 765-8.

[18] Hayward, M. D., Poetgens, A. J., Drewlo, S., Kaufmann, P. & Rasko, J. E. (2007). Distribution of human endogenous retrovirus type W receptor in normal human villous placenta. *Pathology*, *39(4)*, 406-12.

[19] Huppertz, B., Frank, H. G., Kingdom, J. C., Reister, F. & Kaufmann, P. (1998). Villous cytotrophoblast regulation of the syncytial apoptotic cascade in the human placenta. *Histochem. Cell Biol.*, *110*, 495-508.

[20] Janatpour, M. J., Utset, M. F., Cross, J. C., Rossant, J., Dong, J., Israel, M. A. & Fisher, S. J. (1999). A repertoire of differentially expressed transcription factors that offers insight into mechanisms of human cytotrophoblast differentiation. *Dev. Genet.*, *25*, 146-57.

[21] Johnston, J. B., Silva, C., Holden, J., Warren, K. G., Clark, A. W. & Power, C. (2001). Monocyte activation and differentiation augment human endogenous retrovirus expression: implications for inflammatory brain diseases. *Ann. Neurol.*, *50*, 434-42.

[22] Knerr, I., Beinder, E. & Rascher, W. (2002). Syncytin, a novel human endogenous retroviral gene in human placenta: evidence for its dysregulation in preeclampsia and HELLP syndrome. *Am. J. Obstet. Gynecol.*, *186*, 210-3.

[23] Knerr, I., Weigel, C., Linnemann, K., Doetsch, J., Meissner, U., Fusch, C. & Rascher, W. (2003). Transcriptional effects of hypoxia on fusiogenic syncytin and its receptor ASCT2 in human cytotrophoblast

BeWo cells and in ex vivo perfused placental cotyledons. *Am. J. Obstet. Gynecol.*, *189*, 583-8.

[24] Knerr, I., Huppertz, B., Weigel, C., Doetsch, J., Wich, C., Schild, R. L., Beckmann, M. W. & Rascher, W. (2004). Endogenous retroviral syncytin: compilation of experimental research on syncytin and its possible role in normal and disturbed human placentogenesis. *Mol. Hum. Reprod*, *10*, 581-8.

[25] Knerr, I., Schubert, S. W., Wich, C., Amann, K., Aigner, T., Vogler, T., Jung, R., Doetsch, J., Rascher, W. & Hashemolhosseini, S. (2005). Stimulation of GCMa and syncytin via cAMP mediated PKA signaling in human trophoblastic cells under normoxic and hypoxic conditions. *FEBS Lett*, *579*, 3991-8.

[26] Knerr, I., Schnare, M., Hermann, K., Kausler, S., Lehner, M., Vogler, T., Rascher, W. & Meissner, U. (2007). Fusiogenic endogenous-retroviral syncytin-1 exerts anti-apoptotic functions in staurosporine-challenged CHO cells. *Apoptosis*, *12*, 37-43.

[27] Kudo, Y. & Boyd, C. A. (2002). Changes in expression and function of syncytin and its receptor, amino acid transport system B(0) (ASCT2), in human placental choriocarcinoma BeWo cells during syncytialization. *Placenta*, *23*, 536-41.

[28] Kudo, Y., Boyd, C. A., Sargent, I. L. & Redman, C. W. (2003). Hypoxia alters expression and function of syncytin and its receptor during trophoblast cell fusion of human placental BeWo cells: implications for impaired trophoblast syncytialisation in pre-eclampsia. *Biochim. Biophys Acta.*, *1638*, 63-71.

[29] Lavillette, D., Marin, M., Ruggieri, A., Mallet, F., Cosset, F. L. & Kabat, D. (2002). The envelope glycoprotein of human endogenous retrovirus type W uses a divergent family of amino acid transporters/cell surface receptors. *J. Virol.*, *76*, 6442-52.

[30] Lee, X., Keith, J. C. Jr., Stumm, N., Moutsatsos, I., McCoy, J. M., Crum, C. P., Genest, D., Chin, D., Ehrenfels, C., Pijnenborg, R., van Assche, F. A. & Mi, S. (2001). Downregulation of placental syncytin expression and abnormal protein localization in pre-eclampsia. *Placenta*, *22*, 808-12.

[31] Loewer, R., Loewer, J. & Kurth, R. (1996). The viruses in all of us: characteristics and biological significance of human endogenous retrovirus sequences. *Proc Natl Acad SciProc. Natl. Acad. Sci.*, USA., *93*, 5177-84.

[32] Lyden, T. W., Ng, A. K. & Rote, N. S. (1993). Modulation of phosphatidylserine epitope expression by BeWo cells during forskolin treatment. *Placenta, 14*, 177-86.

[33] Malassine, A. & Cronier, L. (2005). Involvement of gap junctions in placental functions and development. *Biochim. Biophys Acta. 1719*, 117-24.

[34] Mangeney, M., Renard, M., Schlecht-Louf, G., Bouallaga, I., Heidmann, O., Letzelter, C., Richaud, A., Ducos, B. & Heidmann, T. (2007). Placental syncytins: Genetic disjunction between the fusogenic and immunosuppressive activity of retroviral envelope proteins. *Proc Natl Acad SciProc. Natl. Acad. Sci.*, U S A, *104*, 20534-9.

[35] Marin, M., Tailor, C. S., Nouri, A. & Kabat, D. (2000). Sodium-dependent neutral amino acid transporter type 1 is an auxiliary receptor for baboon endogenous retrovirus. *J. Virol.*, *74*, 8085-93.

[36] Medstrand, P., van de Lagemaat, L. N. & Mager, D. L. (2002). Retroelement distributions in the human genome: variations associated with age and proximity to genes. *Genome Res.*, *12*, 1483-95.

[37] Mi, S., Lee, X., Li, X., Veldman, G. M., Finnerty, H., Racie, L., LaVallie, E., Tang, X. Y., Edouard, P., Howes, S., Keith, J. C. Jr. & McCoy, J. M. (2000). Syncytin is a captive retroviral envelope protein involved in human placental morphogenesis. *Nature*, *17*, *403(6771)*, 785-9.

[38] Muir, A., Lever, A. & Moffett, A. (2004). Expression and functions of human endogenous retroviruses in the placenta: an update. *Placenta*, *25 Suppl A*, S.16-25.

[39] Nelson, P. N., Hooley, P., Roden, D., Davari Ejtehadi, H., Rylance, P., Warren, P., Martin, J. & Murray, P. G. (2004). Molecular Immunology Research Group. Human endogenous retroviruses: transposable elements with potential? *Clin. Exp. Immunol.*, *138*, 1-9.

[40] Plagemann, A. (2008). A matter of insulin: developmental programming of body weight regulation. *J. Matern Fetal. Neonatal. Med.*, *21*, 143-8.

[41] Peng, X., Pan, J., Gong, R., Liu, Y., Kang, S., Feng, H., Qiu, G., Guo, D., Tien, P. & Xiao, G. (2007). Functional characterization of syncytin-A, a newly murine endogenous virus envelope protein. Implication for its fusion mechanism. *J. Biol. Chem.*, *282*, 381-9.

[42] Pijnenborg, R. (1998). The origin and future of placental bed research. *Eur. J. Obstet. Gynecol. Reprod Biol.*, *81*, 185-90.

[43] Poetgens, A. J., Schmitz, U., Bose, P., Versmold, A., Kaufmann, P. & Frank, H. G. (2002). Mechanisms of syncytial fusion. *Placenta, 23 Suppl A*, S107-13.

[44] Prudhomme, S., Oriol, G. & Mallet, F. (2004). A retroviral promoter and a cellular enhancer define a bipartite element which controls env ERVWE1 placental expression. *J. Virol.*, *78*, 12157-68.

[45] Rasko, J. E., Battini, J. L., Gottschalk, R. J., Mazo, I. & Miller, A. D. (1999). The RD114/simian type D retrovirus receptor is a neutral amino acid transporter. *Proc Natl Acad SciProc. Natl. Acad. Sci.*, U S A., *96*, 2129-34.

[46] Redman, C. W. & Sargent, I. L. (2003). Pre-eclampsia, the placenta and the maternal systemic inflammatory response. *Placenta, 24 Suppl A*, S21-7.

[47] Report of the National High Blood Pressure Education Program Working Group on High Blood Pressure in Pregnancy. (2000) *Am. J. Obstet. Gynecol.*, 183, S1-S22.

[48] Ryan, F. P. (2004). Human endogenous retroviruses in health and disease: a symbiotic perspective. *J. R. Soc. Med.*, *97*, 560-5.

[49] Sacks, G. P., Studena, K., Sargent, K. & Redman, C. W. (1998). Normal pregnancy and preeclampsia both produce inflammatory changes in peripheral blood leukocytes akin to those of sepsis. *Am. J. Obstet. Gynecol.*, *179(1)*, 80-6.

[50] Schreiber, J., Riethmacher-Sonnenberg, E., Riethmacher, D., Tuerk, E. E., Enderich, J., Bosl, M. R. & Wegner, M. (2000). Placental failure in mice lacking the mammalian homolog of glial cells missing, GCMa. *Mol. Cell Biol.*, *20(7)*, 2466-74.

[51] Schubert, S. W., Abendroth, A., Kilian, K., Vogler, T., Mayr, B., Knerr, I. & Hashemolhosseini, S. (2008). bZIP-Type transcription factors CREB and OASIS bind and stimulate the promoter of the mammalian transcription factor GCMa/Gcm1 in trophoblast cells. *Nucleic Acids Res.*, *36*, 3834-46.

[52] Soleymanlou, N., Jurisica, I., Nevo, O., Ietta, F., Zhang, X., Zamudio, S., Post, M. & Caniggia, I. (2005). Molecular evidence of placental hypoxia in preeclampsia. *J. Clin. Endocrinol. Metab.*, *90*, 4299-308.

[53] Sommerfelt, M. A., Williams, B. P., McKnight, A., Goodfellow, P. N. & Weiss, R. A. (1990). Localization of the receptor gene for type D simian retroviruses on human chromosome 19. *J. Virol.*, *64(12)*, 6214-20.

[54] Taruscio, D. & Mantovani, A. (2004). Factors regulating endogenous retroviral sequences in human and mouse. *Cytogenet. Genome Res., 105(2-4)*, 351-62.

[55] Waterstone, M., Bewley, S. & Wolfe, C. (2001). Incidence and predictors of severe obstetric morbidity: case-control study. *BMJ., 322(7294)*, 1089-93.

[56] Yu, C., Shen, K., Lin, M., Chen, P., Lin, C., Chang, G. D. & Chen, H. (2002). GCMa regulates the syncytin-mediated trophoblastic fusion. *J. Biol. Chem., 277(51)*, 50062-8.

[57] Zerangue, N. & Kavanaugh, M. P. (1996). ASCT-1 is a neutral amino acid exchanger with chloride channel activity. *J. Biol. Chem., 271(45)*, 27991-4.

Chapter Sources

The following chapters have been previously published:

Chapter VIII was also published in "Angiotensin Research Progress", edited by Hina Miura and Yuuto Sasaki, Nova Science Publishers. It was submitted for appropriate modifications in an effort to encourage wider dissemination of research.

Chapter IX was also published in "Pregnancy Protein Research", edited by Marie O'Leary and John Arnett, Nova Science Publishers. It was submitted for appropriate modifications in an effort to encourage wider dissemination of research.

Index

A

B

C

D

E

F

G

H

I

J

K

L

M

N

O

P

R

S

T

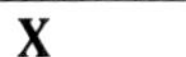
X

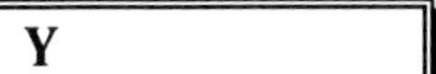
Y

Z